Fitness Nutrition
for
Special Dietary Needs

Stella Lucia Volpe, PhD, RD, LDN
University of Pennsylvania

Sara Bernier Sabelawski, MEd, RD, LDN
University of Massachusetts, Amherst

Christopher R. Mohr, PhD, RD, LDN
Mohr Results

Human Kinetics

Library of Congress Cataloging-in-Publication Data

Volpe, Stella, 1963-
    Fitness nutrition for special dietary needs / Stella Lucia Volpe, Sara Bernier Sabelawski, Christopher R. Mohr.
    p.cm.
    Includes bibliographical references and index.
    ISBN-13: 978-0-7360-4812-5 (soft cover)
    ISBN-10: 0-7360-4812-X (soft cover)
    1. Athletes--Nutrition. 2. Physical fitness--Nutritional aspects. I. Bernier Sabelawski, Sara, 1970- II. Mohr, Christopher R., 1977- III. Title.
    TX361.A8V65 2007
    613.2'024796--dc22
                                                        2006036589

ISBN-10: 0-7360-4812-X
ISBN-13: 978-0-7360-4812-5

The Web addresses cited in this text were current as of February 2007, unless otherwise noted.

Acquisitions Editor: Michael S. Bahrke; **Developmental Editor:** Elaine H. Mustain; **Assistant Editor:** Melissa McCasky; **Copyeditor:** Robert Replinger; **Proofreader:** Erin Cler; **Indexer:** Betty Frizzéll; **Permission Manager:** Carly Breeding; **Graphic Designer:** Fred Starbird; **Graphic Artist:** Dawn Sills; **Cover Designer:** Keith Blomberg; **Photographers (cover):** Left to right: © Human Kinetics, © Human Kinetics, © Photodisc/Getty Images; **Photographer (interior):** All photos (c) Human Kinetics, unless otherwise noted; **Photo Asset Manager:** Laura Fitch; **Visual Production Assistant:** Joyce Brumfield; **Photo Office Assistant:** Jason Allen; **Art Manager:** Kelly Hendren; **Illustrator:** Keri Evans; **Printer:** United Graphics

Printed in the United States of America   10 9 8 7 6 5 4 3 2 1

Human Kinetics
Web site: www.HumanKinetics.com

United States: Human Kinetics
P.O. Box 5076
Champaign, IL 61825-5076
800-747-4457
e-mail: humank@hkusa.com

Canada: Human Kinetics
475 Devonshire Road Unit 100
Windsor, ON N8Y 2L5
800-465-7301 (in Canada only)
e-mail: orders@hkcanada.com

Europe: Human Kinetics
107 Bradford Road
Stanningley
Leeds LS28 6AT, United Kingdom
+44 (0) 113 255 5665
e-mail: hk@hkeurope.com

Australia: Human Kinetics
57A Price Avenue
Lower Mitcham, South Australia 5062
08 8372 0999
e-mail: liaw@hkaustralia.com

New Zealand: Human Kinetics
Division of Sports Distributors NZ Ltd.
P.O. Box 300 226 Albany
North Shore City
Auckland
0064 9 448 1207
e-mail: info@humankinetics.co.nz

I first want to thank God for all of His great gifts. I have dedicated this book to my wonderful husband, Gary R. Snyder; our special German shepherd dogs, Asko and Cenna; my dear parents, Antonio E. and Felicetta Volpe; and siblings, Christina Volpe Lubic, Anthony Volpe, and Loretta Volpe Carter and their families; as well as the Snyder family. My strong family support has helped me throughout my life.

Stella Lucia Volpe

I would like to thank my family, friends, and most of all, my husband, Shawn, for his constant support in all my endeavors. Thanks also to my dear friend and colleague, Stella Volpe, for providing the opportunity to work with her on this project. I would also like to acknowledge my two assistants, Bosco and Zoe, who were always there to give me support.

Sara Jane Bernier Sabelawski

I have dedicated this book to my wife, Kara; my parents, Rich and Linda; and my brother, Kevin. Thank you always for all your love and support and helping make me who I am today.

Christopher R. Mohr

Contents

List of Reproducible Handouts

Reproducible items are identified by the following icon appearing in the outer margin next to them:

Preface

Thank you for buying our book! It will provide you with comprehensive information on nutrition and exercise that you can use to help your clients be at their best when they exercise, whether competitively, for health and fitness, or for recreation. Our goal was to make this an easy-to-use reference for health care professionals who work with athletes. Registered dietitians, sports nutritionists, athletic trainers, personal trainers, physical therapists, sports medicine physicians, and physiatrists all need to be able to provide proper nutrition information to athletes and exercisers with unique dietary needs. This book provides scientifically based information to the health care professional so that he or she can guide clients to eat properly every day for optimal exercise performance at whatever level of exercise they prefer. Coaches will find much of interest in these pages to help them provide sound dietary advice to both the athlete primarily in recreation and fitness and the competitive athlete who wants to achieve optimal performance through improved nutrition.

We have written the text in a reader-friendly style that we hope will make it clear enough to be read and understood by many of your clients with unique needs who exercise. These include athletes and exercisers who are vegetarians, females (with a special focus on pregnant women and postmenopausal women), older adults, children, adolescents, or overweight; athletes who compete in weight-dependent sports; those with disordered eating or diabetes; and those who exercise in very cold or extremely hot and humid weather, or at high altitude. Here are the topics covered in each chapter:

- Chapter 1 focuses on children who exercise and play sports. They are often overlooked because not much research has been conducted on them. People often treat them as little adults, which they are not.

- Chapter 2 discusses older adult exercisers. Not much attention has been paid to this group, either—in terms of their needs for both nutrients and exercise.

- Chapters 3 and 4 concentrate on female athletes and exercisers, with special emphases on menopause and pregnancy, two areas not well written about in the sports nutrition arena.

- Chapter 5 focuses on vegetarian athletes. They are often told that they need to eat meat (especially women), when the focus needs to be on overall energy intake and proper nutrient balance.

- Chapter 6 centers on overweight athletes and exercisers and athletes in weight-dependent sports. With the prevalence of obesity, this chapter is extremely important. Furthermore, most sports nutrition books do not address eating for optimal exercise performance for overweight athletes and exercisers. We realize that not all people are at their ideal body weight, yet many overweight people engage in a structured exercise program.

- Chapter 7 focuses on people who have diabetes mellitus and who exercise. Athletes and exercisers with diabetes mellitus are rarely given information on proper sports nutrition, yet they may have more need for this information than any other group.

- Chapter 8 highlights eating disorders and disordered eating. This chapter covers two main topics: (1) definitions of different types of eating disorders and disordered eating, and (2) ways to provide proper counseling to encourage healthy nutrition and appropriate exercise.

- Chapter 9 discusses the needs of those who exercise in extreme environments such as very cold conditions, hot and humid conditions, or high altitude. Nutritional needs are greater in these conditions, especially for those who exercise for long periods at high intensity.

- The afterword provides a summary, conclusions, and future research recommendations.

The unique features of this book include

- more than 40 reproducibles, including sample meal plans, to hand out to clients or patients: These are listed on pages 7-8 and are also identified by an icon appearing in the outside margin next to each reproducible item,

- in-depth, state-of-the-art scientific information,

- exercise prescription guidelines,

- myths and fallacies about certain topics, and

- case studies written by our guest dietitians and nutritionists that illustrate the practical application of the topic of each chapter.

Each meal plan provided is to be used as a guideline. We recognize that we cannot provide a meal plan for each age, gender, and activity category. Thus, we recommend that you use each meal plan as a base and then adjust it to increase or decrease energy needs, nutrient needs, and so on, depending on the client or patient's age, gender, and activity category. In addition, as for all active people, water consumption throughout the day is important. But people do not need to consume eight 8 oz (240 ml) glasses of water per day because foods and other beverages also provide fluids. Finally, we could not include foods from every country, but the alternative food tables in the appendix can be used in concert with the basic plans to create plans that consider personal food tastes.

We hope that you enjoy this book and that it will become one of your daily reference books. Please let us know how you like the book and how we can improve it for the next edition by contacting Dr. Stella L. Volpe at svolpe@nursing.upenn.edu.

Thanks again for your interest!

Acknowledgments

The authors would like to thank all the dieticians and nutritionists who took the time to provide us with the excellent real-life case studies for each chapter. These certainly added another dimension to this book. We would also like to acknowledge the wonderful people who helped us along the way at Human Kinetics. Though we know that many people were involved, and we thank them, we especially would like to acknowledge Mike Bahrke, our acquisitions editor, who was always so patient; Elaine Mustain, our developmental editor, who guided us, and read through each page so meticulously; Carly Breeding, our permissions manager, who assisted us in acquiring all the permissions needed for this book; and Melissa McCasky, our assistant editor, who worked to complete many loose ends for this book. Without all of your work, this book would have never come to fruition! Thanks again!

Childhood and Adolescence

CHAPTER OVERVIEW

- Nutritional needs
- Major nutritional issues
- Unique nutritional issues for young athletes
- Physical activity
- Case study

This chapter discusses nutrition and physical activity recommendations for children and adolescents. Sources offer various definitions of children and adolescents. According to the Dietary Reference Intake (DRI) tables, children are listed in two categories (because their nutrient needs differ): 1 to 3 years of age and 4 to 8 years of age. Any person age 9 or older is listed as a male or female, with specific subcategories within each grouping: 9 to 13 years of age and 14 to 18 years of age for both males and females. In this chapter, we will use both the DRI definition and the one by Forshee and Storey (2003), which defines children as those 6 to 11 years of age and adolescents as those 12 to 17 years of age. For *nutrient* needs, we will need to refer to the DRI categories, but when we discuss general recommendations for children or adolescents, we will use the Forshee and Storey definition. We will not consider the needs of infants younger than 1 year old.

Like adults, young athletes require sufficient nutrition to perform at their best. Children and adolescents have unique nutritional concerns because they are in the midst of constant physical, mental, and developmental growth. The rapid growth that characterizes infancy tapers off during the years throughout childhood. On average, females experience their most rapid linear growth spurt between 10 and 13 years of age, whereas males experience their rapid growth spurt between 12 and 15 years of age (Shils, 1999). These growth spurts coincide with the years when females and males typically begin puberty; females are usually in the midst of puberty at 12 years of age, whereas males are usually in the midst of puberty a few years later (figure 1.1). The principal health issue regarding children and adolescents is to promote normal growth and development.

Because regular physical activity is an important component of development, energy recommendations and intakes must be adjusted to meet the needs of particular athletic endeavors. Childhood and adolescence can be difficult for parents or caregivers, who are perceived as role models; children and adolescents often pattern their diet and physical activity habits after their parents or guardians. The key is to convey and practice the message of variety, balance, and moderation in food choices to ensure optimal intake for any given physical activity.

Aside from age itself, the primary differences between children and adolescents are the growth spurts and sexual maturation changes that occur during these developmental years. Most noticeable are increases in height, body weight, and the development of secondary sexual characteristics during adolescence. Another physical component of this change is the fluctuation in body

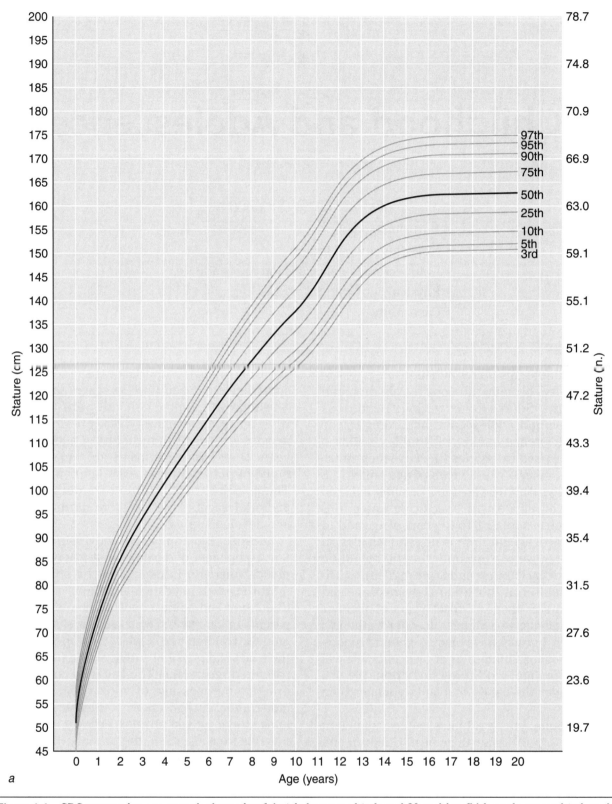

Figure 1.1 CDC stature for age growth charts for *(a)* girls between birth and 20 and for *(b)* boys between birth and 20.

Centers for Disease Control and Prevention, National Center for Health Statistics. CDC growth charts: United States.

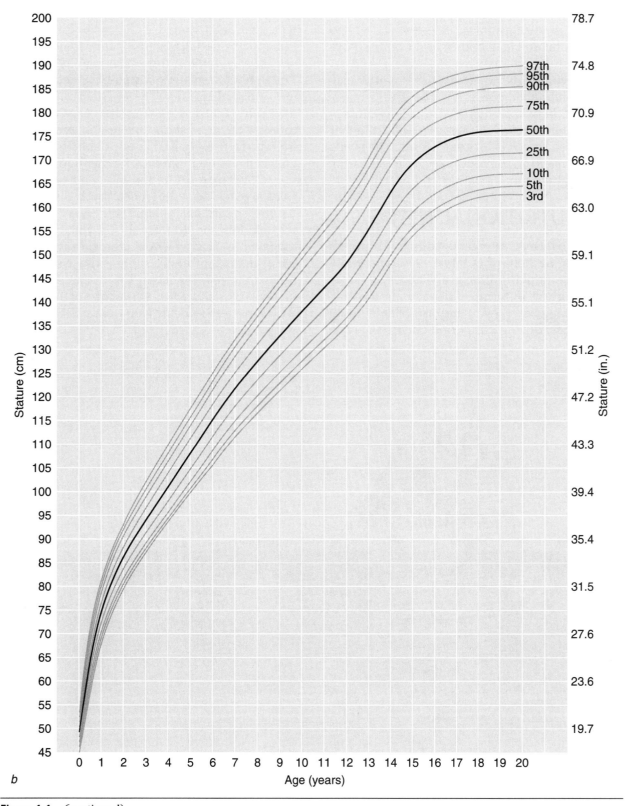

Figure 1.1 *(continued)*

Centers for Disease Control and Prevention, National Center for Health Statistics. CDC growth charts: United States.

composition, which can be particularly important for athletes. During adolescence, females tend to gain body fat and lean body mass, whereas boys gain mostly lean body mass.

Not surprisingly, an increase in appetite usually accompanies growth spurts. The primary difference between children and adolescents is that the number of daily servings will be higher for children than it is for adolescents. The needs of children and adolescents vary little aside from their requirements for energy and protein.

NUTRITIONAL NEEDS

During the formative years of childhood, growth affects eating behaviors. Most children experience large appetite changes. These years are also important in terms of developing the ability to distinguish flavors and establishing food preferences. During this period children may be

categorized as fussy eaters, so planning a well-balanced, nutrient-dense diet can be difficult, but doing so is crucial. Because parents and caregivers are role models, they must lead by example. They should consume a well-balanced, healthy diet and provide children the opportunity to live a healthy, active lifestyle. After children begin to socialize at school, during sports, and with friends, they learn and adopt habits from other children and their parents, further underscoring the importance of the parents' and caregivers' roles in teaching children healthy lifelong habits. Parents, guardians, educators, and other adult role models should introduce a wide variety of foods, emphasizing whole grains, fruits, vegetables, and lean proteins, such as those suggested by MyPyramid, the latest United States Department of Agriculture (USDA) version of the graphic that presents the ideal dietary balance for healthy people of any age (figure 1.2).

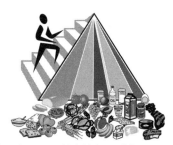

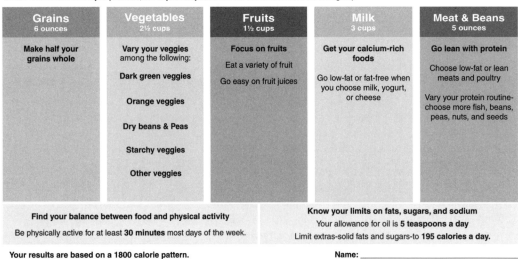

Based on the information you provided, this is your daily recommended amount from each food group

Grains 6 ounces	Vegetables 2½ cups	Fruits 1½ cups	Milk 3 cups	Meat & Beans 5 ounces
Make half your grains whole	Vary your veggies among the following: **Dark green veggies** **Orange veggies** **Dry beans & Peas** **Starchy veggies** **Other veggies**	Focus on fruits Eat a variety of fruit Go easy on fruit juices	Get your calcium-rich foods Go low-fat or fat-free when you choose milk, yogurt, or cheese	Go lean with protein Choose low-fat or lean meats and poultry Vary your protein routine-choose more fish, beans, peas, nuts, and seeds

Find your balance between food and physical activity

Be physically active for at least **30 minutes** most days of the week.

Know your limits on fats, sugars, and sodium

Your allowance for oil is **5 teaspoons a day**

Limit extras-solid fats and sugars-to **195 calories a day.**

Your results are based on a 1800 calorie pattern.   Name: _____

This calorie level is only an estimate of your needs. Monitor your body weight to see if you need to adjust your calorie intake

Figure 1.2   The MyPyramid Web site, found at www.mypyramid.gov, presents the pyramid along with interactive pages that enable users to apply the pyramid to different age groups and to calculate healthy amounts of physical activity for people. The Web site includes material for professionals as well as lay people.

From the United States Department of Agriculture (USDA).
Available: www.mypyramid.gov

The following sections discuss the needs of children and adolescents for energy, macro- and micronutrients, and fluids. But first, we must consider what energy is and how it is measured.

A calorie is a unit of measurement for energy. In most fields, it has been replaced by the joule, the unit of energy used in the International System of Units (SI), but the term *calorie* remains in common use for energy obtained from food. The small calorie, or gram calorie, approximates the energy needed to increase the temperature of 1 g of water by 1 °C. This is about 4.185 joules. Because calories and joules are so small, the common practice when referring to food and energy expenditure is to use the large calorie, or kilogram calorie, which approximates the energy needed to increase the temperature of 1 kg of water by 1 °C. This is about 4.185 kJ, and exactly 1,000 small calories. The term for 1,000 calories is *kilocalories*, abbreviated as *kcal*, and the term for 1,000 joules is *kilojoules*, or *kJ*. Colloquially, and in nutrition and food labeling, the term *calorie* almost always refers to the kilogram calorie.

Energy Needs

Because they are growing and maturing, children have different energy needs than adults do. Physically active children have still greater needs. Active children need enough energy for health and performance as well as for proper growth and maturation. This section focuses on the energy needs of children, especially physically active children.

Energy Needs of Children

Energy needs increase during childhood because of periods of rapid growth and formation of muscle, blood, and bone, which require high levels of anabolic **metabolism**. Because of the rapid changes and fluctuations among children, scientists have noted that specific energy needs are difficult to calculate (Petrie, Stover, & Horswill, 2004; Shils, 1999). Formulas have been derived to estimate a child's energy needs for proper growth and development (*Calculating Energy Requirements for Children,* page 6). In addition, the DRI for Estimated Energy Requirements (EERs) for children 6 to 11 years of age (in this case, EERs are calculated, so we used the Forshee and Storey [2003] definition of children) are approximately 1,793 and 1,758 kcal per day for girls 6 and 11 years of age, respectively, and 2,088 and 2,038 for boys 6 and 11 years of age,

respectively. Note that these are approximations, because activity levels and body weight and height are all taken into account. Refer to the DRI tables for **macronutrients** to calculate specific energy needs for children (www.iom.edu/Object.File/Master/21/372/0.pdf).

Of course, physical activity plays a large role in the energy requirements and needs of children. Those who are sedentary will require significantly less energy than their more active counterparts who participate in activities such as playing with friends, riding bikes, or playing organized sports. Although using the aforementioned formulas would be more accurate, the National Center for Health Statistics (NCHS) growth charts are a simple way of tracking general nutrition and energy adequacy by following growth patterns over time.

Energy Needs of Adolescents

As it does in children, physical activity plays a major role in the energy requirements of adolescents. Estimating the energy needs of an adolescent is difficult because of the rapid physical changes that occur during these years. The most important consideration is to consume adequate energy. Adolescents should eat until satisfied to fulfill their needs; however, this does not mean he or she should overeat. Portion control is one important method of preventing weight gain.

The EERs for adolescents are approximately 1,751 and 1,716 kcal per day for girls 12 and 17 years of age, respectively; and 2,028 and 1,978 kcal per day for boys 12 and 17 years of age, respectively. Be aware that these numbers will fluctuate depending on the activity level of the person. Again, refer to the DRI table for more accurate calculations based on energy expenditure and age (www.iom.edu/Object.File/Master/21/372/0.pdf).

Other Nutritional Needs

The importance of adequate hydration cannot be overemphasized, especially because children are generally unable to tolerate temperature extremes as well as adults do (Steen, 1996b). Water should be the primary fluid consumed, but skim milk is also an important fluid because it provides an excellent source of vitamins and minerals, like calcium and vitamins A and D. The intake of soda and sweetened drinks should be discouraged because these products provide a

Calculating Energy Requirements for Children

One method of calculating energy requirements for children is the following.

For boys 3 to 8 years of age use this formula:

$$88.5 - (61.9 \times \text{age}) + (\text{PA} \times [26.7 \times \text{body weight} + 903 \times \text{height}]) + 20^\S$$

For girls 3 to 8 years of age use this formula:

$$135.3 - (30.8 \times \text{age}) + (\text{PA} \times [10.0 \times \text{body weight} + 934 \times \text{height}]) + 20^\S$$

In both formulas, PA = physical activity. You should calculate

- age in years,
- body weight in kilograms, and
- height in meters.

Other factors to take into account follow.

Boys

- If the child is sedentary, use 1.00 for PA.
- If the child is low active, use 1.13 for PA.
- If the child is active, use 1.26 for PA.
- If the child is very active, use 1.42 for PA.
- For boys 9 through 18 years of age, replace 20 with 25.

Girls

- If the child is sedentary, use 1.00 for PA.
- If the child is low active, use 1.16 for PA.
- If the child is active, use 1.31 for PA.
- If the child is very active, use 1.56 for PA.
- For girls 9 to 18 years of age, replace 20 with 25.

For calculating the activity level of the child, use these criteria:

- Sedentary = no activity.
- Low active = active for about 30 to 60 minutes per day.
- Active = active for about 60 to 90 minutes per day.
- Very active = active for more than 90 minutes per day.

$20^\S$ is a constant used in energy requirement equations for boys and girls.
Formulas from G.M. Wardlaw, J.S. Hampl, and R.A. DiSilvestro, 2004, *Perspectives in nutrition*, 6th ed. (Boston, MA: McGraw-Hill Higher Education).

high amount of energy with very few nutrients (see table 1.1). Although 100% fruit juices are good sources of nutrients and fluids, even these should be limited because many children and parents do not think about the high kilocalorie content of these juices when calculating the appropriate amount of food to consume. Children and adolescents should be encouraged to eat more whole fruits and decrease the consumption of 100% fruit juices to one or two servings (6 oz, or 175 ml) per day. Whole fruits also provide fluid and fiber.

The DRI for water has been established as an Adequate Intake (AI) as follows: 1.7 liters (L) per day for children 4 to 8 years of age (boys and girls); 2.1 and 2.4 L per day for girls and boys, respectively, 9 to 13 years of age; and 2.3 and 3.3 L per day for females and males, respectively, 14 to 18 years of age. Note, however, that these needs change with heat, humidity, and activity levels; that foods provide about 20% of water needs each day; and that beverages other than water can help to meet these recommendations (see *Calculating Daily Fluid Requirements*, on page 7).

Calculating Daily Fluid Requirements

100 milliliters (ml) per kilogram (kg) for the first 10 kg of body weight

+ 50 ml per kg for the next 10 kg of body weight

+ 20 ml for every kilogram of body weight over 20 kg

Examples of minimum daily fluid intake:

For 9 kg child: 9 kg × 100 ml = 900 ml

For 12 kg child: (10 kg × 100 ml) + (2 kg × 50 ml) = 1,100 ml

For 29 kg child: (10 kg × 100 ml) + (10 kg × 50 ml) + (9 kg × 20 ml) = 1,680 ml

Conversions:

1 L = 1,000 ml

1 L = 35.28 oz of water

1 L = 33.8 fluid oz

1 cup = 8 fluid oz

1 kg = 2.2 lb

Formula from Health Canada, 2002, *Fluid management: Fluid requirements in children*. (Online). Available: www.hc-sc.gc.ca/fnih-spni/ pubs/nursing-infirm/2001_ped_guide/chap_04_e.html#4-1.

Although all nutrients play important roles in the diet, specific macro- and micronutrients are of utmost concern. Protein needs are elevated during childhood and adolescent years when anabolic metabolism is high, especially during growth spurts. Similarly, three minerals in particular are vital for optimal growth: Calcium is necessary for proper bone mineral density deposition, iron is essential for blood cell formation, and zinc is important in hormone production and skeletal and muscle formation. The United States Department of Agriculture (USDA) MyPyramid provides adequate nutrition guidelines for children and adolescents. As with adults, the serving requirements from MyPyramid must meet the needs of children and adolescents and be balanced with regular physical activity.

Most health professionals are already aware of these general guidelines. More important is being able to assess nutrient deficiencies and nutrient overdoses. Obviously, the biggest nutrient "overdose" today is the overconsumption of total energy, leading to overweight and obesity. This condition is often a result of malnutrition (*malnutrition* means "bad nutrition," not just undernutrition but overnutrition as well). And even an overweight child or adolescent may be deficient in nutrients because of poor eating habits. Table 1.1 describes signs of nutrient deficiencies that you should be familiar with. When performing a nutrition assessment with a child or

Table 1.1 Signs of Nutrient Deficiencies

Appearance	Nutrient deficiencies
General appearance of apathy; muscle or tissue wasting; excessive irritability; underweight, undersized, and underdeveloped for age; paleness and loss of color of the skin, nail beds, lips, or hair; spoon-shaped nails (iron)	Protein, energy, thiamin, niacin, riboflavin, iron, zinc
Hair that is dry, wiry, stiff, brittle, easily pulled out, very red, or has lost color	Protein, zinc
Nails that are spoon-shaped (iron), brittle, ridged, cracking	Iron, vitamin C
Skin that cracks, flakes, or scales; irregular pigmentation; fluid retention and edema; dermatitis; small hemorrhages or bruises	Protein; essential fatty acids; vitamins A, K, and C; niacin; riboflavin; or iron
Eyes that are small, circular, grayish or yellowish gray, dull, or dry; foamy irritations on the surface of the eye; inflammation of the eyelids; softening or thickening of the outer surface of the eye; loss of night vision or ability to adapt from dark to light	Vitamin A, riboflavin, or iron
Face that has irritations at the corners of the mouth, greasy scaling around the nose or mouth, cracking around the mouth	Protein, riboflavin, or iron
Mouth that is smooth, reddened, shiny, or swollen; dry tongue; swollen or bleeding gums; excessive tooth decay; reduced taste sensation	Vitamin C, niacin, riboflavin, folate, or vitamin B$_{12}$

From S.L. Volpe, S.B. Sabelawski, and C.R. Mohr, 2007, *Fitness nutrition for special dietary needs* (Champaign IL: Human Kinetics).
Adapted from www.mamashealth.com/nutrition/defi.asp.

adolescent, having one of the parents or guardians present would be helpful, but it would also be a good idea to talk with the child and caregiver separately, if possible, because you will be able to obtain more information. Children and adolescents often have a difficult time changing their dietary habits because they typically depend on their parents or guardians. Some children or adolescents, however, prepare meals for themselves or the household, an additional important piece of information. Behavior change is the key, so learning about what the particular client does is the first step in knowing what behaviors to work on changing first.

Nutrient needs also depend on gender, age, and activity level. For example, the older a person becomes, the lower his or her energy needs are. Males require more overall energy than females do because of greater muscle mass (on average). The higher a person's activity levels are, the greater his or her energy needs are. The next sections discuss each of these nutrient needs.

Carbohydrate

As outlined in the USDA MyPyramid, carbohydrate should be the mainstay of the diet for sedentary children and athletes alike. Complex carbohydrates are necessary for optimal physical performance and energy, but most importantly as fuel for the brain. It is not clear, however, whether young athletes benefit from a high-carbohydrate diet as adult athletes do. This is most likely because children are thought to lack full development of glycolytic capacity (Eriksson, 1972). On the contrary, it appears that this lack of development disappears during adolescence, suggesting that young athletes would benefit from a higher-carbohydrate diet (Eriksson). Therefore, all young athletes should consume approximately 50% of their daily energy intake

from carbohydrate. If your client has accepted the popular low-carbohydrate diet myths, you will find material to help you address this issue in chapter 6.

Both the quantity and quality of carbohydrate intake are important. Carbohydrate should be grain-based, high-fiber foods that provide a multitude of vitamins, minerals, and other important nutrients. Foods such as whole-grain cereals, vegetables, fruits, pasta, potatoes, and legumes are great choices. With children, emphasize grain-based snacks rather than high-sugar, low-nutrient snacks, because children derive a significant portion of total energy from snacks. Refer to table 1.2, which gives examples of good versus poor carbohydrate choices. You can photocopy it to give to your clients or their parents.

Protein

In accordance with the Dietary Reference Intakes (DRI), children (4 to 13 years of age) should consume approximately 0.95 g of protein per kg of body weight per day (Food and Nutrition Board [FNB], 2005). A 28 kg child would therefore need approximately 27 g of protein per day, an amount that is easily obtained from a varied diet with adequate energy intake. Little is known about the effects of regular physical activity on protein needs and utilization in children (Rodriguez, 2005). In adults we know that exercise increases protein needs, but the little information available for children makes it difficult to make specific recommendations. Health practitioners must rely primarily on estimates (Bolster, Pikosky, McCarthy, & Rodriguez, 2001). Pikosky, Faigenbaum, Westcott, & Rodriguez (2002) suggested that the downregulation of protein metabolism observed in the exercising children in their study might be more of an energy intake issue rather than solely a protein concern. More research in this area is

Table 1.2   Examples of Poor Versus Better Carbohydrate Choices

Poor carbohydrate choice	Better carbohydrate choice
Peanut butter sandwich on white bread	Peanut butter sandwich on whole-wheat bread
Sugar-coated corn flakes cereal	Regular corn flakes cereal
White pasta and sauce	Wheat pasta blend and sauce
Chocolate-covered granola bar	Whole-grain granola bar

From S.L. Volpe, S.B. Sabelawski, and C.R. Mohr, 2007, *Fitness nutrition for special dietary needs* (Champaign, IL: Human Kinetics).

clearly warranted. This conclusion reemphasizes the importance of the recommendation that children meet their energy needs by consuming nutrient-dense foods to ensure healthy physical and mental growth.

The DRIs for protein in adolescents are actually lower than those for children because of the lower growth rate during adolescence compared with childhood. Sedentary adolescents (14 to 18 years of age) should consume approximately 0.85 g of protein per kg of body weight per day (FNB, 2005).

Refer to table A.1 in the appendix (page 159), which lists protein sources that should be selected most often, moderately often, and least often. You may photocopy this table and give it to your clients.

Fat

Dietary fat is a crucial component of development. The focus in this food group should be on healthy fats, like olive oil, fish, and nuts rather than saturated and trans fats that are found in butter, most snack foods, and whole-fat dairy products. Children and adolescents should consume approximately 25% of their total energy from fat. Table A.3 (page 160) summarizes typical fat sources that should be used most often, moderately, and least often.

Vitamins and Minerals

Vitamins and minerals are also important to growth, development, and athletic performance in children and adolescents. Because the scope of this book does not permit discussion of all *micronutrients*, we will discuss only calcium and iron at length.

• **Calcium.** Calcium intake is crucial at a young age to ensure adequate development of bone mineral density. Although the effects of chronic low calcium intake are not usually apparent until adulthood, inadequate intake may lead to stress fractures. However, calcium is not the only important factor in bone health. Total energy intake, protein intake, and vitamin D intake all

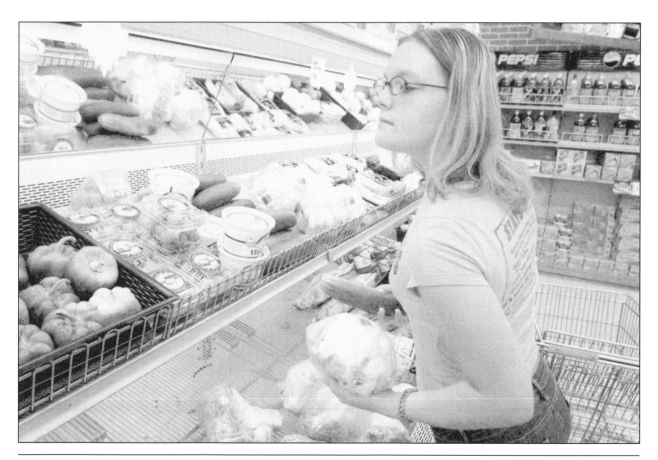

A parent can empower herself to shop wisely at the grocery store for her children's health if she takes the time to learn about their unique nutritional requirements.

play a role in bone strength. Therefore, calcium supplementation should not be suggested across the board. Instead, ensure adequate energy intake from a variety of foods, particularly those that are quality sources of calcium, such as dairy products (milk and yogurt, for example), dark leafy green vegetables, and certain nuts (almonds, for example).

• **Iron.** Inadequate iron intake can have an acute effect, leading to iron deficiency *anemia*. Chronic low iron intake may lead to lower stores of iron, which affect muscle metabolism, cognitive function, and could lead to fatigue (Bar-Or, IOC Medical Commission, & International Federation of Sports Medicine, 1996; Grantham-McGregor & Ani, 2001). Iron intake should be monitored with the onset of menses in young women and subsequent increase in blood loss. Similarly, iron deficiency anemia sometimes appears in boys during their growth spurts. Moreover, besides losing blood through menses, females may restrict their energy intake because of concern with body image, a common issue with young female athletes. This restriction in energy may mean a decrease in food variety from potentially highly bioavailable *heme* sources of iron, like animal protein. Heme iron, the more easily absorbed form of iron, is mostly found in animal protein like red meat, poultry, and fish. Nonheme iron is derived from nonanimal protein and is not as readily absorbed because these foods are usually bound to an organic constituent of that food, making it less available. Cooking often breaks these bonds and makes the iron more available, but heme iron is still more easily absorbed than nonheme iron. Concomitant consumption of quality sources of vitamin C, such as orange juice, however, increases the absorption of nonheme iron (Hallberg, 1981). If a person is restricting dietary sources of iron, iron supplementation is not necessarily warranted unless a true deficiency of this mineral is present. Quality sources of iron include, but are not limited to, red meat, green leafy vegetables, enriched grains, iron-fortified products (cereal, whole grains, rice, macaroni, and so forth), legumes, and dried fruits.

• **Other minerals and vitamins.** Because a plethora of information is available about vitamins and minerals, we suggest that you refer to any basic nutrition book and to the Dietary Reference Intake books, each of which will provide information on nutrient deficiencies, excesses,

and needs for children and adolescents. Also refer to table 1.1 (page 7), which describes micronutrient deficiencies. Note that each child or adolescent has specific needs based on his or her frequency and intensity of exercise, dietary intake, and growth rate. Being specific with children and adolescents who exercise or who are athletes is even more important, because growth and development also need to be factored into the equation. Recall that you can photocopy and provide table 1.2 (page 8) to parents or adolescents about healthy snack choices and the nutrients that they provide.

MAJOR NUTRITIONAL ISSUES

Ensuring that a child or adolescent consumes a proper balance of foods that matches his or her energy expenditure is imperative for optimal exercise performance and growth and development. The next sections highlight some areas regarding proper energy balance.

Importance of Breakfast

After children enter school, their eating patterns become more scheduled, thus reducing the risk of deficiencies. Typically this period is characterized by few feeding problems because of the availability of different foods and food programs for children from all socioeconomic backgrounds. Breakfast foods are of particular importance; several studies have made a connection between breakfast consumption and enhanced cognitive performance (Bellisle, 2004; Pollitt & Mathews, 1998). In addition, youngsters who eat breakfast typically consume about 200 to 500 more kcal per day and have higher intakes of other nutrients than those who do not consume breakfast (Nicklas, Bao, Webber, & Berenson, 1993; Sampson, Dixit, Meyers, & Houser, 1995).

In addition, most breakfast foods are cereal or grain based, meaning that they are high in carbohydrate and often low in fat. This kind of diet is important not only for optimal mental function but also for restoring liver glycogen stores for sustained energy. Furthermore, ready-to-eat breakfast cereal is fortified with a number of vitamins and minerals. An additional benefit is that ready-to-eat cereals are typically consumed with dairy products such as skim milk or yogurt, thus increasing calcium intake.

Sample Meal Plans for Children and Adolescents

Each meal plan provided is to be used as a guideline. We cannot provide a meal plan for each age, gender, and activity category, so you should use the meal plan as a base and then adjust upward or downward to meet energy and nutrient needs, depending on age, gender, and activity category. In addition, as for all active people, water consumption throughout the day is important. Children and adolescents need not consume eight 8 oz (240 ml) glasses of water per day because foods and other beverages also provide fluids. Also, note that the metric measures included are close approximations rather than exact equivalents. Finally, we realize that we could not include foods from every country; but we hope that these meal plans will provide a guide for foods from other countries that are similar in energy and nutrients. See tables A.1 through A.4 in the appendix for alternative protein, carbohydrate, and fat sources and a list of fruits and vegetables sorted by kind of vitamin and micronutrient provided.

Children

Breakfast

- 1/2 cup of oatmeal = 30 g
- 1/2 cup of low-fat milk = 120 ml
- 1/2 of a medium banana = 65 g
- 1/4 cup of raisins = 3 g
- 1/2 cup of orange juice = 120 ml

Snack

- 2 oz of animal crackers = 54.4 g
- 1 oz of string cheese = 28 g
- 8 oz of water = 240 ml

Lunch

- 2 tbsp of natural peanut butter = 30 g
- 2 tbsp of 100% fruit jelly = 30 g
- 2 slices of whole-wheat bread = 80 g
- 1/2 cup of baby carrots = 4 g
- 1/2 cup of low-fat milk = 120 ml
- 4 oz of water = 120 ml

Snack

- 1/2 cup of applesauce = 1.5 g
- 6 to 10 small whole-wheat cracker squares = 100 g
- 8 oz of water = 240 ml

Dinner

- 1 cup of spaghetti with marinara sauce = 500 g
- 1/2 cup of broccoli = 4 g
- 1 whole-wheat dinner roll = 80 g
- 1 cup of mixed greens salad = 30 g
- 1 tbsp of salad dressing of choice = 15 g
- 1/2 cup of low-fat milk = 120 ml
- 4 oz of water = 120 ml

Snack

- 1/2 cup of pudding of choice = 1.5 g
- 1 cup of fresh strawberries = 166 g
- 8 oz of water = 240 ml

This sample meal plan provides at least 100% of the Dietary Reference Intakes (DRIs) for energy, protein, *fiber,* vitamins A, C, E, B_6, B_{12}, thiamin, riboflavin, niacin, folate, calcium, iron, magnesium, phosphorus, and zinc and approximately

- 2,000 kcal (8,360 kJ),
- 60 g of protein,
- 50 g of fat,
- 25 g of fiber, and
- 2,441 mg of sodium.

Adolescents

Breakfast

- 1 cup of whole-grain cereal (Raisin Bran, Cheerios, oatmeal, and so on) = 60 g
- 1 cup of skim milk = 240 ml
- 1/2 of a medium banana = 65 g
- 1/2 cup of orange juice = 120 ml

Snack

- 1/4 cup of mixed nuts = 5 g
- 1/2 cup of dried fruit = 6 g
- 8 oz of water = 240 ml

Lunch

- 2 slices of whole-wheat bread = 80 g
- 2 oz of sliced turkey breast = 50 g
- 1 slice of cheese of choice = 25 g
- 1 tbsp of mustard = 15 g
- 1 medium orange = 120 g

(continued)

Sample Meal Plan *(continued)*

- 1/2 cup of skim milk = 120 ml
- 4 oz of water = 120 ml

Snack

- 1 cup of baby carrots = 8 g
- 1 oz of string cheese = 28 g
- 6 small whole-wheat cracker squares = 80 g
- 8 oz of water = 240 ml

Dinner

- 3 oz of grilled chicken breast = 90 g
- 1 medium sweet potato = 130 g
- 1 cup of mixed greens salad = 30 g
- 1 tbsp of salad dressing of choice = 15 g
- 1 whole-wheat dinner roll = 80 g
- 1/2 cup of skim milk = 120 ml
- 4 oz of water = 120 ml

Snack

- 1 cup of plain or vanilla low-fat yogurt = 220 g
- 1/2 cup of fresh or frozen blueberries = 20 g
- 1/4 cup of granola = 20 g
- 8 oz of water = 240 ml

This sample meal plan provides at least 100% of the Dietary Reference Intakes (DRIs) for energy (kilocalories), protein, fiber, vitamins A, C, E, B_6, B_{12}, thiamin, riboflavin, niacin, folate, calcium, iron, magnesium, phosphorus, zinc, and approximately

- 2,300 kcal,
- 110 g of protein,
- 74 g of fat,
- 37 g of fiber, and
- 2,600 mg of sodium.

From S. L. Volpe, S.B. Sabelawski, and C.R. Mohr, 2007, *Fitness nutrition for special dietary needs* (Champaign, IL: Human Kinetics).

Clearly, then, breakfast is important for optimal physical and mental growth, particularly for athletes, whose energy needs are higher than those of their sedentary counterparts. Performance will suffer if a child or adolescent does not consume adequate energy. The old adage that breakfast is the best way to start the day is true. Moreover, it has been reported that people of all ages who eat breakfast burn approximately an additional 55,000 kcal per year on average, so emphasizing the importance of breakfast is crucial.

Snacks

Snacks provide a good portion of the nutrient intake of school-age children and adolescents. Snacks contribute up to one-third of their total energy intake (Nicklas, 1995). In dual-income households, children and adolescents often prepare their own snacks. Having a variety of convenient, nutrient-dense, and tasty snacks on hand will provide another opportunity for children and adolescents to increase their energy and nutrient intake. Table 1.3 provides a suggested list of snack foods and some nutrients that they provide. You may photocopy this table for your clients and their parents.

Although caregivers are often concerned that children or adolescents snack too often, snacking is not an unhealthy practice if the snacks consumed are nutrient-dense foods rather than sugary snacks that may also be high in fat. This concern is particularly important for young athletes and physically active children whose nutritional needs are higher. Snacking provides additional energy throughout the day, helping to fuel children's bodies and minds. In fact, because a child's stomach is rather small, offering smaller meals and snacks throughout the day may reduce the risk of overeating and still provide the necessary energy and nutrition. Nonetheless, the importance of healthy snacking must be emphasized. A la carte and vending machines in schools are often places where children can find less healthy snacks. Although schools (and many states) are trying to change what is offered in a la carte and vending machines, children need to be taught that healthy snacking is the best for their growth, cognitive function, and athletic performance. This guideline does not mean that children can never have a sweet snack, but most of the time they should choose healthier foods—those that are nutrient dense but not energy dense.

Table 1.3 Healthy Snack Options

Food choice	Sample of nutrients and benefits
Fresh raw vegetables	Vitamins A and C, antioxidants
Low-fat yogurt	Calcium, vitamin D, protein
Dried fruit	Iron, vitamins A and C, antioxidants
Mixed nuts	Healthy fats, protein, vitamin E
Canned soup	Variety of vitamins and minerals, depending on type
Fresh fruit	Filling, low-energy source of vitamins A and C, antioxidants
Trans fat free, whole-grain crackers	Complex carbohydrates, fiber, B vitamins
Ready-to-eat cereals (low sugar)	Iron, calcium, complex carbohydrates
Popcorn	Fiber, carbohydrate
Low-fat cottage cheese and fruit	Convenient; variety of nutrients, depending on specific type of fruit
Whole-grain bread, peanut butter and jelly	Fiber, carbohydrate, healthy fat, convenient

From S.L. Volpe, S.B. Sabelawski, and C.R. Mohr, 2007, *Fitness nutrition for special dietary needs* (Champaign, IL: Human Kinetics).

Overweight and Obesity

In 2004 the *Journal of the American Medical Association* (*JAMA*) released statistics of at risk for overweight and overweight in U.S children and adolescents. In 2002 31.5% of children 6 through 19 years of age were at risk for overweight and 16.5% were overweight (Hedley et al., 2004). Defining at risk for overweight and overweight is not as simple with children and adolescents as it is with adults, for whom the **body mass index (BMI)** is useful. BMI is calculated with this formula:

$$BMI = weight \ (kg) \ / \ height \ (m^2).$$

The *JAMA* article defined at-risk for overweight as at or above the 85th percentile but less than the 95th percentile of the sex-specific BMI for age. This condition is defined by growth charts and identifies children who may be at risk for being overweight, but a second screening is required to determine the next step in the intervention, if any (See BMI charts in the appendix on pages 161-162). Overweight was defined as at or above the 95th percentile of the sex-specific BMI for age.

A physical exam or other intervention, such as assessment of body composition, would be necessary to determine whether the child is truly overweight (i.e., overfat). This step is particularly important with athletes. Body composition can be used as a measurement tool to track changes over time if a qualified healthcare professional performs the measurements (Steen, 1996b). The **bone mineral density** and proportion of body water in children differ greatly from those of adult athletes, so standardizing body composition values is difficult. Although methods to determine body composition to account for these differences exist (Deurenberg, van der Kooy, Paling, & Withagen, 1989; Houtkooper, Lohman, Going, & Hall, 1989), using body fat as a screening criterion for sports participation or setting weight requirements for younger athletes is not recommended (Steen). The concern is that setting such weight requirements could negatively affect growth and development. Nonetheless, assessing body composition in young athletes may establish that they indeed have more muscle and not more fat, thus decreasing the chances that they will be identified as being overweight.

Childhood and adolescent overweight affects short- and long-term physical and mental health. In the short term, children who are at-risk for overweight or overweight are often teased and ridiculed, causing embarrassment, a decrease in self-esteem, and sometimes depression. Over the long term, obesity can have severe health consequences, such as ***cardiovascular disease***

Myths About Children and Weight Loss

Some believe that overweight children need to go on a "diet." Granted, some children are morbidly obese and may require severe measures to decrease their body weight so that they can preserve their health. Nonetheless, for the child who is overweight or at-risk for overweight, a change in dietary intake, which often leads to a decrease in energy intake, is what should be emphasized. That is, a child needs to eat foods that are higher in **nutrient density** and lower in energy density to promote growth and prevent obesity. A child also needs to be physically active daily. Incorporating physical activity is not that difficult. Families can even exercise together when they are watching television. During commercials, each family member must think of an activity (for example, sit-ups, push-ups, dancing) that the family must do together. This approach turns a sedentary behavior into a physically active, family-interactive behavior! A child may then use this method when he or she is watching television alone. Furthermore, the entire family can become more active by incorporating fun, vigorous activities into the family routine by walking, swimming, cycling, playing ball, or another activity.

(CVD), type 2 **diabetes mellitus (DM)**, and **hypertension**. Although these health concerns do not typically appear until adulthood, chronic diseases begin in childhood and manifest themselves in adulthood. Furthermore, type 2 diabetes mellitus, which until recently manifested itself only in adults, has become more prevalent in younger children. This dramatic rise in type 2 diabetes mellitus is due almost entirely to the rise in obesity (Fagot-Campagna, 2000; Ludwig & Ebbeling, 2001). In fact, a publication in the *New England Journal of Medicine* suggests that the current trend toward extended longevity in youth today will quickly reverse itself if the rise in obesity and its related health consequences continues (Olshansky et al., 2005). Moreover, scientists suggest that unless the obesity epidemic is reduced, younger people will lead less healthy and shorter lives than their parents did (Olshansky et al.).

The only way to reduce overweight and obesity and the subsequent negative health outcomes is to decrease overall energy intake moderately and increase levels of physical activity. Because the energy guidelines fluctuate with children and adolescents, a one-size-fits-all energy requirement cannot be established. Consuming lower-fat food items, particularly foods with less saturated fat and trans fat, and decreasing the intake of high-sugar, high-fat drinks, snacks, and foods is a general way to improve the quality of the diet without limiting growth and development or causing a detriment to athletic performance.

All children and adolescents should also be encouraged to be more active in general. Although organized sports can be beneficial, they should not be the only channel for increasing physical activity. Families need to limit computer and television time; television watching has been linked to the development of obesity (Klesges, Shelton, & Klesges, 1993). Although the environment is not the sole cause of the obesity epidemic, anything that takes away from opportunities to be more physically active (television, computer, and so forth) is a contributor. Children and adolescents need to be shown by example that regular physical activity and healthy eating are fundamental to leading a long, healthy life.

What usually works best for overall behavior change in children is a change in the behavior of the entire family. Usually, but not always, the child has become overweight because of the family's habits, not just his or her habits. Thus, the entire family should make a pact to become healthier—to eat healthier, to be more physically active, and to take time to be together as a family. These times together help build confidence in children. Families can cook together as well, an activity that helps children learn the importance of cooking healthily and using fresh ingredients. Being creative can help all family members change their behavior and lead a healthier lifestyle.

To help avoid overweight and obesity in the first place, children should not be forced to eat or to clean their plates, as many parents encourage them to do. Research has shown that infants and young toddlers have the innate ability to self-regulate energy intake (Fox, Devaney, Reidy, Razafindrakoto, & Ziegler, 2006). Parents and guardians need to be educated not to diminish these cues by telling children to clean their plates, because coercive feeding can lead children to lose their ability to regulate their eating as they

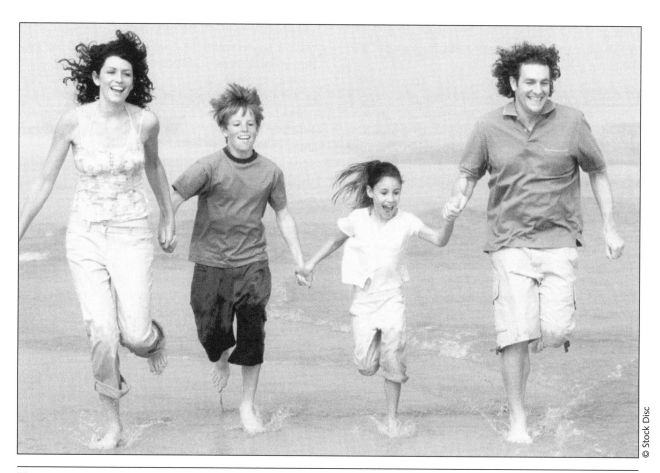

© Stock Disc

The most effective strategy for helping overweight children to incorporate more physical activity into their lives is for parents to promote physical activity for the entire family, including themselves. Engaging in active recreation together is a great first step.

get older. Similarly, overrestriction of intake can lead to overeating later in life (Fox et al.).

This ability is often distorted when environmental cues and outside influences encourage children, for example, to clean their plates or eat more of their dinner if they expect to eat dessert. These practices may lead children to eat when they are not hungry, to ignore their natural hunger cues, and to lose their ability to distinguish between physiological hunger and psychological hunger. This circumstance may lead to overweight and obesity.

Of course, a pediatrician and a registered dietitian should monitor weight-loss practices to ensure that growth and maturation are not negatively influenced. Another important point to consider is that the more positive tactic of ensuring controlled weight gain in a child may decrease the chances of putting the child at risk for deficiencies during growth. This recommendation may be most appropriate for children in the 85th to 94th percentile on the BMI growth charts, those classified as at risk for overweight (Hedley et al., 2004), rather than those at or above the 95th percentile, who are classified as overweight.

Rather than promoting a drastic reduction in foods or food groups, a more healthy practice would be to encourage variety, balance, and moderation in food choices to ensure that a child is obtaining the proper nutrition. The snack ideas in table 1.3 may help a child establish healthy eating patterns that will enhance the nutrient content of the diet and thereby limit the possibility of having nutrient deficiencies.

Body Image

Discussing all associated behaviors, practices, and health effects of eating disorders is beyond the scope of this chapter, so we will touch on them only briefly. For an in-depth discussion, see chapter 8 on disordered eating. For even more detail, we suggest reading *Disordered*

Eating Among Athletes: A Comprehensive Guide for Health Professionals by Katherine Beals, PhD, RD (Beals, 2004).

As children grow older, body image often becomes a major concern. Because of the rapid physical growth and body development in adolescence and the common struggle with identity, body image concerns and eating disorders are more common among this age group than any other. This is a concern with adolescent females in particular, but it can also be an issue with children and adolescent males. One-half to three-quarters of all adolescent females report a history of dieting. Unfortunately, adolescents who report a history of dieting are also more likely to have a poor body image and indulge in unhealthy practices such as fasting, vomiting, taking diet pills, and binge eating (Littleton & Ollendick, 2003; Moore, 1993). This concern is also common in weight-sensitive and aesthetic sports, such as wrestling, ballet, figure skating, swimming, and diving. Athletes in these sports often diet to meet the requirements or desires of their coaches rather than make healthy choices for their bodies. Coaches, referees, judges, and teammates need to be sensitive to the fact that a single comment can lead to an eating disorder. All should know the signs and symptoms of eating disorders. Please refer to chapter 8 on eating disorders within this text for further information.

Inadequate Nutrition

Although children and adolescents in North America rarely show clinical signs of malnutrition, some consume diets that are inadequate in quantity, quality, or both. In particular, the intake of protein, calcium, iron, zinc, and vitamins A, C, and B_6 is sometimes below recommended intakes, the latter three in nonathletic children in particular (Kennedy & Goldberg, 1995). Although clinical deficiencies such as scurvy may not be present, growth and maturation could be affected.

Undernutrition may have serious consequences for younger people. Inadequate and unbalanced nutrition can lead to fatigue, dehydration, disordered eating, impaired growth, and increased risk for infection and illness. Poor nutrition may also prevent a child from participating fully in learning experiences (Steen, 1996a). Moreover, research has demonstrated that although the intake of certain vitamins and minerals may be low, the intake of dietary fat, sodium, and sweets often is not. When a child underconsumes nutrient-dense foods and relies heavily on sweets and high-fat items, his or her growth may be negatively affected.

Fortunately, the school-age period is one of relatively steady growth and few apparent feeding problems. As previously discussed, many school systems now offer breakfast in addition to the normal lunch offerings. Many parents shun school meals for their apparent nutrition inadequacy, but research has demonstrated that home-packed lunches provide significantly fewer nutrients than school lunches do, although they do offer less **saturated fat** (Ho et al., 1991). This is not to say that home-packed lunches are poor choices for parents; obviously, the nutritional quality of the lunch depends on what foods, snacks, and beverages are included in it. The options for home-packed meals are limited by the lack of refrigeration, so parents must read food labels and make sound decisions about what nonperishable foods would provide well-balanced meals. In addition, the analyses of school lunch nutrients do not include a la carte items that may be high in saturated fat, energy, and sodium, skewing the data from the earlier mentioned study (Ho et al., 1991).

Nutrition education should be stressed during childhood and adolescence. Children and adolescents will be making innumerable choices. Parents and educators must provide a sound nutrition foundation so that kids can ultimately make choices that positively affect their health. For children, nutrition is crucial as they attempt to master physical and mental skills throughout the day. Likewise, adolescents face problems as they go through puberty. Peer pressure has a strong influence on most young people during these years, so they must develop healthy eating and physical activity habits early. Many strategies can be used to instill good habits in children and adolescents. Role modeling tends to be the most effective way for children to learn good health habits, although not all children of physically active parents are physically active. But if parents practice healthy habits, their children are more likely to do so as well. Teaching children and adolescents why it is important to be healthy is also an effective method. Knowledge is powerful, and providing information to children and adolescents about healthy eating and exercising can be quite successful.

UNIQUE NUTRITIONAL ISSUES FOR YOUNG ATHLETES

In this section, we will highlight the unique needs of young athletes, including weight-control issues and fluid and nutrient needs. All are important for the proper growth and optimal performance of young athletes and exercisers. Young athletes must realize that eating and hydrating properly are just as important to achieving their goals as working out is.

Weight Control

Adolescents, in particular adolescent girls, seem to be prone to weight-control issues such as disordered eating. In this section, we discuss weight-loss practices in athletes, as well as the female athlete triad. For an in-depth look at disordered eating and eating disorders, refer to chapter 8.

Weight-Loss Practices

Sound nutrition and activity guidelines cannot be disregarded in pursuit of achieving an athletic goal. Rapid weight-loss practices are most common in weight-classification sports (wrestling, crew) and sports that emphasize aesthetics (gymnastics, diving, figure skating, ballet). Acutely, these dangerous weight-loss practices can lead to dehydration, fatigue, weakness, and injury. Chronically, dangerous weight-loss practices like fasting, food and fluid restriction, or attempting to increase sweating by wearing a rubber suit while training in a steam room may result in nutrient deficiencies, eating disorders, impaired growth, or in extreme cases, death. During this period of growth and maturation, drastically restricting energy intake through a reduction or elimination of foods or food groups is unwise. To maintain health and fitness, males should have a body-fat level of at least 7% and females should have a body-fat level of at least 14% (Oppliger, Case, Horswill, Landry, & Shelter, 1996). Young athletes and their coaches need to be aware of these figures.

Female Athlete Triad

The female athlete triad is composed of three components: disordered eating, *amenorrhea*, and osteoporosis (figure 1.3). Disordered eating was discussed earlier and appears to the under-

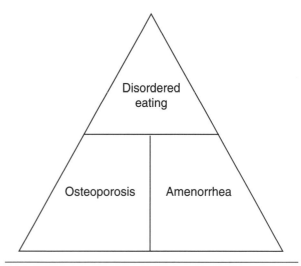

Figure 1.3   The female athlete triad is not a trivial syndrome. On the contrary, it can be life threatening. For detailed information on approaching and helping girls with the triad, see chapter 8.

lying behavior for the female athlete triad (see chapter 8 for more information). Amenorrhea is the absence of menses, often referred to as athletic amenorrhea. The true cause of athletic amenorrhea is not clearly understood, but it is believed to result from energy balance disturbances that may be a result of poor food choices, an extreme reduction in energy intake, or excessive exercise and training practices. The last component of the female athlete triad is osteoporosis, which literally means "porous bones." Most people think that osteoporosis is a disease that affects only older women or elderly people, but disordered eating or amenorrhea can lead to osteoporosis. In this situation, some physicians may prescribe oral contraceptive pills to counter hormonal imbalances, and they may recommend calcium supplementation to prevent continued resorption (breakdown) of the bones.

From a dietary perspective, each athlete needs individual help in making the positive changes necessary to prevent more serious medical issues from arising. For some girls with the female athlete triad, a team approach may be needed if the disordered eating is severe (for example, an eating disorder). Thus, a registered dietitian, physician, psychologist, social worker, and the female athlete would need to work together. The female athlete triad can be a difficult condition to tackle because many athletes are happy not to menstruate because they believe that menstruating negatively affects performance. Thus, athletes need to be educated on the negative consequences of amenorrhea. In particular, learning how the female athlete triad can affect performance rather than learning that it is harmful to her health is more likely to induce a young woman to change her energy intake and training practices. A step-by-step approach is needed to help an athlete recover. The main things to focus on are energy intake and exercise training, although tackling one of these at a time usually produces better results.

Fluid and Nutrition Needs

Fluid and nutrition are both important for maintaining health and peak performance. In this section, we focus on the needs of the young athlete or exerciser for fluid, macronutrients, and micronutrients.

Fluid and Hydration

Training improves the ability to thermoregulate, which allows athletes to acclimate more quickly than the unfit person can. But this does not mean that the athlete needs less fluid than the nonathlete, or that he or she needs less fluid in the heat. Optimal fluid intake is an important component of health and performance. A decrease in body weight of as little as 1%

through exercise-induced sweating negatively affects endurance performance (Wilk, Yuxiu, Bar-Or, Wouters, & Saris, 2002). Adequate fluid balance is important not only for performance but also for cardiovascular and thermoregulatory function.

Although plain water is the best source of fluid for activity under 60 minutes in duration, sports drinks may enhance hydration status and performance for activities lasting longer than 60 minutes that are performed in the heat (Convertino et al., 1996). In addition, if heat is an issue, a sports drink will replace the additional electrolytes lost because of increased sweating. Moreover, sports drinks or diluted fruit juice may be more palatable than water for children, increasing the likelihood of regular consumption. Children prefer flavored carbohydrate-electrolyte drinks to water, and this, in turn, can prevent voluntary dehydration in trained young athletes who are exercising in a hot environment but are already acclimatized to the heat (Rivera-Brown et al., 1999). Like adults, children should not wait until they are thirsty to consume fluids; they should consume fluids before, during, and after exercise.

Energy Needs

Young athletes and physically active children have energy needs greater than those of their more sedentary counterparts to compensate

---

What Are Electrolytes?

Electrolytes are a group of minerals—sodium, potassium, and chloride—that are important to fluid balance. In some cases, bicarbonate is included, because it acts as a buffer. Electrolytes are minerals that become ions in solution, and in doing this, they obtain the ability to conduct electricity. Blood levels of these electrolytes are measured to assess whether a person is within the normal range. The role of electrolytes in the body is important, so maintaining a normal range is important.

- Sodium is the primary positive ion (also known as a cation) that is located outside the cells. Sodium combined with chloride is known as table salt. Sodium has many roles, but one of them is to regulate the total body water. A normal blood range for sodium is 125 to 145 millimoles per liter (mmol per L).
- Working in conjunction with sodium is potassium, which is the major positively charged ion inside the cells. Potassium is required in the body for normal heart rhythm and muscle contraction. Normal blood potassium concentrations range from 3.5 to 5.0 mmol per L.
- The primary negatively charged ion (anion) is chloride, which is located in the extracellular fluid. The normal blood levels for chloride range from 98 to 108 mmol per L.
- The main role of the bicarbonate ion is to buffer blood levels to preserve normal pH levels at 7.4. Normal blood levels of bicarbonate range from 22 to 30 mmol per L.

for the energy expenditure from the activity. To ensure proper growth and maturation, children must consume adequate total energy and nutrients. As noted earlier, however, establishing a DRI for children is difficult because of the large variability in activity levels and growth rates (Petrie et al., 2004). Moreover, different populations (obese children versus elite athletes) tolerate the stress of exercise differently, and energy expenditure calculations may underestimate actual needs. Therefore, guidelines can serve as a baseline for intake needs, but children should be monitored individually to determine whether the intakes are adequate to meet their needs and demands. The growth charts in the appendix are a good starting point for children. If a child is maintaining normal growth patterns for his or her height and age, there should not be concern. In addition, the formulas in the section *"Calculating Energy Requirements for Children"* (page 6) can serve as a guideline for determining energy needs.

Other Nutrients for Athletic Performance

Although we touched on nutrient needs earlier in the chapter, the following sections briefly discuss how nutrients can affect athletic performance.

• **Protein**. Most young athletes in developed countries are not at risk for protein deficiency. Although sufficient protein is necessary for growth and repair, there is little concern if a child is consuming enough total energy. Inadequate energy intake will cause protein to be used inefficiently to provide energy to lean tissues, rather than being used to synthesize, rebuild, and repair lean tissue. Because little information is available about the protein needs of adolescent athletes, the most important consideration in this population is not protein intake but total energy intake. If a young athlete or exerciser does not consume enough energy, a protein deficiency or protein-energy malnutrition can occur. If this condition becomes severe, signs and symptoms include dry, brittle, or even wiry hair; brittle nails; cracks around the mouth; apathy; edema or swelling around joints and, in particular, around the abdomen area; and fatigue.

• **Fat**. Dietary fat plays an important role in exercise performance. Petrie et al. (2004) have even suggested that it may be as important as

carbohydrate. Dietary fat is essential for hormone production, for protection of the viscera and central nervous system, and for energy. The type of fat that a person consumes is what is important. Although people should consume 20% to 30% of their total energy intake from fat, the highest percentage of that intake should be derived from **monounsaturated fat** (olive oil, avocados, flaxseeds and oil, peanut butter, and so forth). Although young athletes do not typically connect their current eating habits to chronic disease later in life, athletes should be taught that diseases like heart disease begin not at age 50 but at a young age.

• **Vitamins and minerals**. Earlier in the chapter, we suggested that nonathletic children often have inadequate intakes of certain vitamins and minerals, even though their energy intake is high through consumption of high-sugar and high-fat foods. Fortunately, studies have suggested that young athletes are less likely to underconsume their daily requirements for vitamins than their nonathletic peers are (Rankinen, Fogelholm, Kujala, Rauramaa, & Uusitupa, 1995). Research has not established that physically active children (and adults) require greater intakes of vitamins and minerals, but some studies have shown that transient changes occur after exercise with some minerals and that a deficiency could ensue over time. Currently, however, the evidence is not strong enough for health professionals to tell athletes to consume vitamins and minerals above the DRI. But young female athletes, in particular adolescents, may require higher calcium and iron intakes because of the greater risk of **osteoporosis** later in life and to menstruation, respectively (Lytle, 2002).

Dietary Supplements

Typically, the appeal of dietary supplements is not as influential among children and adolescents as it is with adults, but parents may extrapolate what they hear and read for themselves and feel that supplementation is warranted if their child is an athlete. Despite the widespread interest in supplements, research does not support the notion that vitamin and mineral supplements will enhance growth, development, performance, or mental function in well-nourished athletes (Haymes, 1991). Because athletes have higher energy requirements and subsequently consume a greater amount of food, they are typically able to meet their increased needs through the diet.

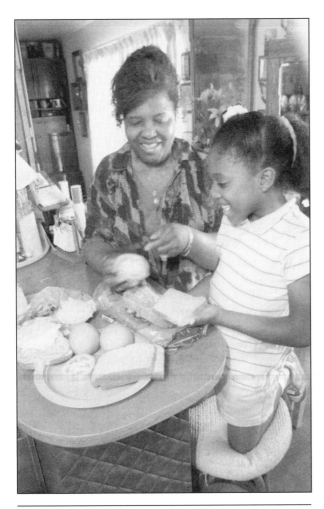

One way parents can instill good eating habits in their children is to make fixing healthy food a fun activity they can do together.

This approach should be adequate unless a true clinical deficiency is diagnosed, at which time it is important to take the advice of a pediatrician and registered dietitian.

PHYSICAL ACTIVITY

Children and adolescents who do not regard themselves as athletes should be encouraged to increase their physical activity and exercise regularly. Children should be taught that exercise helps the body remain healthy and strong. As appropriate for their age, they can learn that exercise assists with

- strengthening the heart, lungs, and circulatory system;
- helping to control appetite;
- helping to maintain body weight;

- increasing levels of **high-density lipoprotein cholesterol (HDL-C),** which removes cholesterol from the blood before it enters the wall of the artery;
- decreasing levels of **low-density lipoprotein cholesterol (LDL-C),** which carries cholesterol to the artery walls; and
- maintaining energy balance and allowing a higher intake of food, which increases the likelihood of consuming a well-balanced diet.

Strategies for Helping Children Be Active

Many people assume that children are more active than adults because they are constantly on the go. Unfortunately, as the overweight and obesity epidemics continue to increase, this belief is untrue. Children are increasingly occupying their time with TV and computers, and engaging in other sedentary behaviors rather than moving their bodies.

Regular physical activity and exercise do not have to be synonymous with organized team sports. Although beneficial for many young people, team sports may intimidate and discourage other children from getting any regular exercise. Moreover, children who are not among the better athletes on the team may not be involved enough to move their bodies and obtain the health benefits of exercise. Children can be active in other ways, and regular playtime needs to be encouraged. Physical activity means moving the body and getting the heart and muscles working. The 2005 USDA dietary guidelines suggest that children and adolescents should engage in at least 60 minutes of physical activity on most, preferably all, days of the week. In addition, the Institute of Medicine released several new recommendations (Koplan, Liverman, & Kraak, 2005), including the following:

- Schools should ensure opportunities for students to accumulate 30 minutes of moderate to vigorous physical activity each day.
- The food and beverage industry should implement guidelines about marketing and advertising to children.
- Parents need to provide healthy foods at home, like fruits and vegetables, and encourage their kids to choose them as snacks.

- Parents should encourage physical activity by limiting sedentary activities, like television and computer time.

The recommendations for adolescents are similar to those for children. The primary difference between the age groups is that adolescents undergo various growth and development phases, particularly during puberty as growth spurts occur, as appetites and attitudes change, and as more options become available. Parents or guardians must become involved. They must educate their children and lead by example by eating a balanced diet and engaging in regular physical activity.

Exercise Prescription Guidelines

The most important exercise guideline for children and adolescents is to be active on all or most days of the week. Children should accumulate at least 60 minutes and up to several hours of age-appropriate physical activity on those days. The activity can be anything that they enjoy—bike riding, playing tag with friends, playing hopscotch, jumping rope, and so on. Any activity that gets the body moving is acceptable. Many children, especially younger children, will not get excited about riding on a stationary bicycle or walking on a treadmill. For the most part, children enjoy spontaneous games, running and playing, and levels of high intensity followed by levels of lower intensity (which equates to interval training). Physical activity does not have to occur through organized sports. Simply going outside and playing with friends, just moving the body, may be the best kind of activity.

Children should participate in an extended period of physical activity. Parents and guardians should discourage their children from sitting in front of the TV or computer for more than 2 hours at a time.

CASE STUDY

Although this chapter has focused on the child and adolescent athlete, the combination of eating a healthy diet, engaging in an adequate amount of exercise, and maintaining a healthy body weight has been a thread that runs through this chapter. As we stated in the preface, we were fortunate to have several dietitians provide us with real-life case studies of their clients that we can share with our readers. We hope that these case studies will provide you with some new ideas to use in your practice. The case study in this chapter focuses on an overweight child. Read on to see what our guest dietitian provided.

The client is a 9-year-old male who entered our weight-management program in October 2004 with significant weight gain in the past 6 months (20 lb, or 9.1 kg). His beginning height and weight were 54.5 in. (138.4 cm) and 151 lb (68.6 kg). His mother is a single mom who works 10-hour shifts 4 to 5 days per week, making it challenging for her to cook and make nutritious meals. The hectic lifestyle required her to rely on fast food for afternoon snacks and dinner. After school, the client stayed at his grandparents' house, where meals were prepared in traditional Southern style (heavy cream sauces, high-fat meats, and large portions). From there, his mother picked him up when she finished working.

His lifestyle included limited physical activity and many hours of participation in video games and television.

Typical Food Intake Before Entering the Program

A 3-day record of the client's food consumption before he entered the program indicated that he was eating on average 3,200 kcal (13,376 kJ) per day (plus or minus 300 to 500 kcal, or 1,254 to 2,090 kJ). He engaged in physical activity only 1 day per week during physical education class at school (for about 45 minutes).

Breakfast—7:00 a.m.
- 2 Pop Tarts or 2 bowls of Cocoa Puffs with whole milk
- 12 oz of apple juice (360 ml)

School lunch—12 noon

(3 days per week; meals varied depending on menu cycle)

- Hamburger, hot dog, or hot meal (red beans, rice, sausage, fruit, french fries or Tater Tots, bread or roll)
- Milk

After-school snack—4:00 p.m.
- Happy Meal from McDonald's with regular soda
- Potato chips and soda, or candy bar and soda (convenience store)

Dinner—7:00 p.m.

- Fast food 2 to 3 days per week—Happy Meal or Value Meal from McDonald's, depending on hunger level
- Home meals—5 to 6 oz (150 to 180 g) of high-fat meat (sausage or fried chicken), breaded and fried fish, or, occasionally, baked or grilled meat
- Side dishes—baked macaroni with cheese (1 to 1 1/2 cups), rice and gravy (3/4 cup), one or two slices of bread (80 to 160 g)
- Vegetables—typically corn or peas, occasionally green beans or broccoli
- Fluids—12 to 16 oz (360 to 480 ml) of juice or punch

Snack—8:30 p.m.

(one of the following only if hungry, 3 to 4 days per week)

- 1 cup (220 g) of yogurt
- 1/2 cup (110 g) of regular ice cream
- Bag of popcorn (salted, buttered)

Exercise Modifications

The client began a combination of strength and cardiovascular training 3 days per week for 1 hour each session. Exercise consisted of circuit training on youth machines, spin classes for kids, and functional circuit training using his body weight. The local YMCA offered this program, which was affordable for this single parent, who had a limited income. Many schools have free after-school programs, which could be another option for families who have a limited income.

Nutrition

One of my goals was to avoid requiring the mother or the child to count kilocalories (or kilojoules) because they already had difficulty managing their schedule. I focused initially on establishing three nutrition goals that would

1. reduce fluid kilocalorie intake to less than 100 kcal per day (418 kJ per day),
2. increase frequency of eating more nutrient-dense snacks and more fiber, and
3. promote smarter choices at breakfast and when dining out, specifically fast food.

Revised Food Intake

Breakfast—7:00 a.m.

(choose one of the following)

- 2 whole-grain Eggo Waffles with 1 tbsp (15 g) of peanut butter on each
- 1 cup of cereal (1/2 cup of Cocoa Puffs, 1/2 cup of Kashi Heart to Heart) (220 g) with 8 oz (240 ml) of 1% milk
- Smoothie (8 oz, or 240 ml, of skim milk; 2 tbsp, or 30 g, of Ovaltine; 1 medium banana or fruit of choice (80 g); and 1 tbsp (15 g) of peanut butter

School lunch—12 noon

On days when the school offered a high-fat or fried option (hot dog, hamburger, or pizza), I let him pick his favorite option and recommended that his mother pack a bagged lunch for him to take to school the other 2 or 3 days. The bagged lunch recommendation was the following:

- Deli sandwich (lean turkey, ham, or tuna) or peanut butter and jelly (100% Simply Fruit or Polaner All Fruit) on whole-wheat bread, fresh fruit or cup of fruit packed in juice
- 100 kcal (418 kJ) snack pack or yogurt (less than 100 kcal, or 418 kJ, per serving)

After-school snack—4:00 p.m.

I provided a list of healthy snack options for children to his mother and grandparents for after-school snacks.

Dinner—7:00 p.m.

- When they did eat at fast-food restaurants, I instructed the child and his mother to use a fast-food handout that I provided, which lists the energy content of foods at those restaurants.
  - Have a small hamburger or grilled chicken sandwich; hold the mayonnaise or sauce other than mustard or ketchup (no more than 2 tsp, or 10 g, total).
  - Substitute salad with 2 tbsp of a vinaigrette dressing for french fries, or his mother can bring fresh fruit.
  - Substitute low-fat milk for soda.

- Home meals—lean meats such as chicken, fish, lean ground beef (no more than 4% fat), or extra-lean ground turkey (4 to 5 oz, or 120 to 150 g) grilled, broiled, or baked.
- Side dishes and starches—1/2 to 1 cup of whole-grain pasta, 1 to 2 slices of wheat bread, 1 cup of corn or peas, or small baked potato (60 to 120 g, 80 to 160 g, 110 g, respectively).
- Vegetables—1 to 2 cups (60 to 120 g) of broccoli with 1 slice (30 g) of fat-free cheese or light parmesan cheese.
- Fluids—water or very low kilocalorie juices (for example, diet V8 Splash).

Snack—8:30 p.m.

(one of the following only if hungry, 3 to 4 days per week)

- 6 oz (100 g) of yogurt, less than 100 kcal (418 kJ) per serving, or 1/2 cup (60 g) of light or low-fat ice cream (no sugar added)
- 1 cup (80 g) of light microwave popcorn

A follow-up with 3-day food records indicated that energy intake was approximately 1,800 to 2,200 kcal (7,524 to 9,196 kJ) per day with much higher energy expenditure than previously noted. His exercise bouts increased to 4 to 5 days per week instead of only 1 day per week during physical education class. He continued to participate in the 3-month weight-management program for two more sessions (for a total of 6 months) and made continued progress.

Overall Accomplishments

This particular 9-year-old boy was motivated and achieved a great deal during this time. His accomplishments included

- improved eating habits (lower energy and sugar intake, more nutrient-dense foods, portion control, and improved hydration),
- increased exercise frequency and level of physical fitness, and
- lower body weight and waist circumference.

In 6 months, this boy was able to decrease his body weight by 20 lb (9.1 kg), from 151 lb (68.6 kg) to 131 lb (59.5 kg), thus losing the body weight that he had gained. He also decreased his waist circumference by 4 in. (10.2 cm). He increased in height by 0.5 in. (1.3 cm) over the 6 months. At 12 months, he grew another inch (2.5 cm) and decreased his body weight by another 5 lb (2.3 kg). I continue to monitor him every other month to ensure that he is growing properly and managing his body weight in a sensible way.

Tavis Piattoly, MS, RD
American College of Sports Medicine Certified Health and Fitness Instructor
Training and Wellness Program Manager, Elmwood Fitness Center
Director of Nutrition, Tulane University Athletics New Orleans, Louisiana

Aging

America is an aging society. The United States Census Bureau (www.census.gov/prod/www/abs/popula.html) estimates that in the year 2030, approximately 20% of the United States population will be 65 years of age or older. Chronological age, however, is a poor predictor of health. With the increase in the number of healthy and active people toward the upper end of this age spectrum, research has suggested that we need additional definitive age groups, such as the young old, age 65 to 75; the old old, age 75 to 85; and the oldest old, those older than age 85. Likewise, with life expectancy at a record high of about 77 years for the general population in North America, people should strive to live not only longer but also healthier.

Nutrition and exercise, two of the chief determinants of successful aging, play a major role in increasing the number of healthy years and decreasing the number of years with illness. Of course, aging is a complex process that involves a number of variables, such as genetics, lifestyle, and chronic disease. Leading a healthy lifestyle and extending the number of healthy years can lead to what is referred to as the compression of *morbidity*. Now, more than ever, people are interested in turning back the clock to slow the aging process. Unfortunately, body cells age no matter what lifestyle we lead. Research has shown, however, that a number of factors can help modify longevity in adults. Several lifestyle factors were identified in centenarians and correlated to their longevity (Johnson, Brown, Poon, Martin, & Clayton, 1992):

- Consume fruits and vegetables regularly
- Consume a large amount of whole grains
- Perform daily physical activity
- Eat breakfast
- Consume a small amount of saturated fats
- Drink alcohol only in moderation
- Do not smoke
- Gain little weight in adulthood

The thought of a long life is wonderful, but only if our health does not fail as we age. Quality of life is at least as important as quantity.

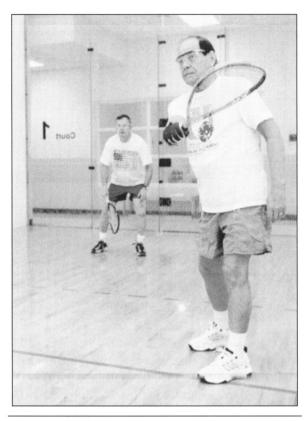

These gentlemen have found a way to simultaneously increase their health, promote their social life, and have fun.

PHYSIOLOGICAL CHANGES IN AGING

Several biological changes that occur with aging affect dietary needs. The onset and extent of these changes are different for each person, so predicting when or to what extent they will occur in all older adults is impossible.

- Less stomach acid is produced, which could decrease the absorption of vitamins B_{12} and C.
- A natural decrease occurs in **lean body mass**, meaning that energy needs decline.
- Up until physical maturity, the **anabolic** processes (growth factors) exceed the **catabolic** processes (breakdown) of body cells (for example, lean tissue and other internal cells). After the body reaches physiologic maturity, the balance between anabolic and catabolic processes shifts and the catabolic, or degenerative, mechanisms prevail.

- The skin naturally produces less vitamin D, increasing the dietary requirements for this vitamin, which is crucial for bone health, a major concern in the aging population, particularly women.
- Older adults have a decrease in thirst sensation, increasing the risk of dehydration.
- Sight, hearing, smell, and taste sensitivity may all decline with age (Schiffman, 1997); the latter two may increase the likelihood that a person will consume an inadequate diet (Bilderbeck, Holdsworth, Purves, & Davies, 1981).

Although a healthy diet and regular physical activity cannot prevent any of these changes from occurring, they may be able to slow their development or progression.

NUTRITION

Most researchers have focused their attention on the prevention of chronic disease through a healthful diet. As more research emerges, it is apparent that the best diet for older adults is one that is balanced with whole grains, plenty of fruits, lean proteins (emphasizing fish), and plant proteins (for example, nuts). Undoubtedly, good nutrition throughout life is a clear factor in determining the quality of life that a person may expect in later years. Besides observing the general recommendation to consume a balanced diet, older adults can refer to a food guide pyramid created by Tufts University that emphasizes particular nutrients of concern to older people (figure 2.1). Specific dietary recommendations for the older population are different from those for the general population because of the physiological and functional changes discussed previously.

Energy Needs

Obesity is an epidemic, and its **comorbidities** are associated with a shortened life span, particularly for morbidly obese women and moderately obese men because of their body-weight distribution. Similarly, some data have shown that being underweight is associated with a **mortality** rate as high as that seen in obesity in those over 60 years of age. What, then, should a person believe?

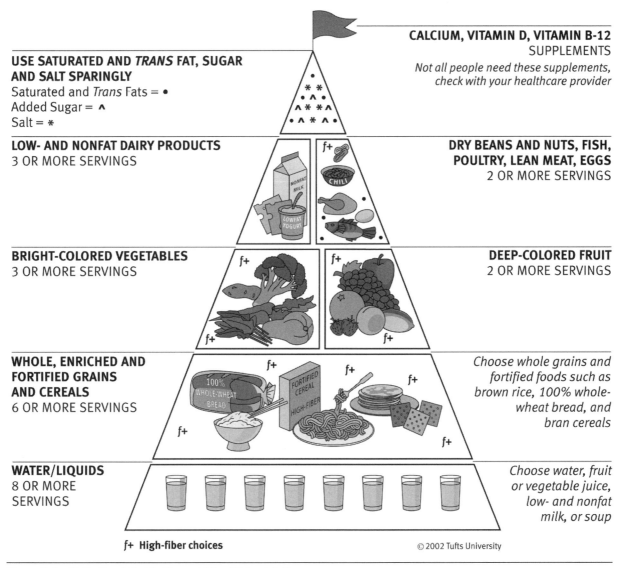

CALCIUM, VITAMIN D, VITAMIN B-12
SUPPLEMENTS
Not all people need these supplements, check with your healthcare provider

USE SATURATED AND *TRANS* FAT, SUGAR AND SALT SPARINGLY
Saturated and *Trans* Fats = •
Added Sugar = ∧
Salt = *

LOW- AND NONFAT DAIRY PRODUCTS
3 OR MORE SERVINGS

DRY BEANS AND NUTS, FISH, POULTRY, LEAN MEAT, EGGS
2 OR MORE SERVINGS

BRIGHT-COLORED VEGETABLES
3 OR MORE SERVINGS

DEEP-COLORED FRUIT
2 OR MORE SERVINGS

WHOLE, ENRICHED AND FORTIFIED GRAINS AND CEREALS
6 OR MORE SERVINGS

Choose whole grains and fortified foods such as brown rice, 100% whole-wheat bread, and bran cereals

WATER/LIQUIDS
8 OR MORE SERVINGS

Choose water, fruit or vegetable juice, low- and nonfat milk, or soup

f+ **High-fiber choices**   © 2002 Tufts University

Figure 2.1   Tufts Food Guide Pyramid for Older Adults.

From S.L. Volpe, S.B. Sabelawski, and C.R. Mohr, 2007, *Fitness nutrition for special dietary needs* (Champaign, IL: Human Kinetics).

• **We know that energy requirements decrease with age**. These changes come primarily from the natural loss of lean body mass and subsequent increase in fat mass. Physical inactivity decreases energy needs even further, not only because of the decrease in energy output but also because less physical activity will cause greater loss of lean body mass. Therefore, people must remain physically active to slow the loss in lean body mass that occurs naturally with aging. By consuming a wide variety of nutrient-dense foods and engaging in regular physical activity, older adults can slow these losses of lean body mass.

• **We do not fully understand the relationship between energy restriction and longevity**. Although the practice of restricting energy intake to increase life span is becoming more common, the number of people who are adopting this type of diet is relatively small and its practice is still controversial. Although more than 70 years of evidence from animal studies indicates that those on decreased energy diets may be able to extend their life span, we have no direct scientific evidence for humans. Regardless, many have extrapolated the findings from animals and adopted them into their lives. The landmark study in this area of work was conducted in the 1930s, when a researcher found that energy intake regulates the rate of growth and the rate and development of aging. In this particular study, the researcher fed rats a diet that was adequate in all the necessary vitamins, minerals, and protein but was limited in total energy. As the researcher added energy, the animals began to grow and mature. The animals whose diets were limited in total energy lived twice as long as those that consumed the "normal" diet with no energy restrictions. In animals on energy-restricted diets, detrimental age-related changes in physiologic function are prevented, delayed, or reduced dramatically. In addition, the development of chronic disease appears to be slowed. A number of theories have been advanced about why this decrease in energy intake may be correlated to increased life span in animals, but more research is needed to prove these theories. Moreover, we do not know whether the increased life span in animals will extrapolate to an increased life span and improved quality of life in humans.

The most reasonable recommendation at this stage, then, is to strike a balance between a moderate energy restriction (to match the natural decrease in lean body mass) and regular physical activity. Such a balance appears to promote the positive health benefits observed in energy-restricted animals.

Other Nutritional Needs

In this section, we focus on macronutrients, fiber, some vitamins and minerals, and fluid needs of the older adult. These items are all important for people to consider as they age, especially those who exercise. Teaching older people to read food labels is important because many "hidden" items, such as salt, may need to be decreased in an older person's diet. Refer to figure 2.2 for an example of food labels, what they must include, and how to educate people to interpret them.

Protein

In the United States, protein intake is usually not an issue for most age groups. But the older adult who has drastically decreased his or her energy intake will often reduce protein intake as well, increasing the risk of protein malnutrition or protein energy malnutrition. The Dietary Reference Intakes (DRI), established as a Recommended Dietary Allowance (RDA) for adults, is 0.8 g of protein per kg of body weight per day. One study published in the mid-1990s suggested, however, that protein intake of 1.0 g per kg per day is more appropriate for the aging population to maintain nitrogen balance (Campbell, Crim, Dallal, Young, & Evans, 1994). Another group of researchers reported that increased protein intake above normal levels may have a favorable effect on bone mineral density in older men and women (Dawson-Hughes, Harris, Rasmussen, Song, & Dallal, 2004). This slight increase in needs most likely results from decreased efficiency in protein utilization. The greatest concern with this population is maintaining a nutrient-dense, energy-balanced intake. Protein deficiency is rare in older Americans unless they have some type of debilitating disease, but protein is still a crucial nutrient in helping to heal body tissues (particularly with regular exercise) and maintain a strong immune system, because immune responses normally decline with age.

Carbohydrate

As seen in the Tufts Food Guide Pyramid for Older Adults in figure 2.1, the number of servings of grain products is only 6, compared to the 6 to 11 servings recommended in the USDA food guide pyramid for adults. (Note: The recent release of MyPyramid recommends 5 to 6 oz [150 to 180 g] of grain, depending on age and physical activity versus the six servings recommended in the Tufts Food Guide Pyramid.) The decrease in the amount of carbohydrate and grain-based foods accompanies the overall decrease in total energy needs for older adults. The recommended amount of carbohydrate and grain-based foods is also smaller because reduced glucose tolerance is common among older adults, particularly those who are inactive (Ryan, 2000). Moreover, the key with carbohydrate intake is not quantity, but quality. Complex carbohydrates, such as those derived from whole grains, supply more fiber, vitamins, and minerals, all of which may be in shorter supply with lower energy intake and a less varied diet.

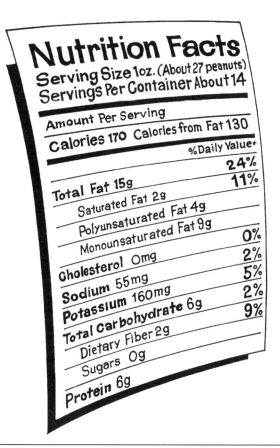

Figure 2.2 This example of a food label shows what it must include and how it can be used to educate people. The nutrition facts label explains quantities of each nutrient on food labels that are desirable (see table 2.1).

From S.L. Volpe, S.B. Sabelawski, and C.R. Mohr, 2007, *Fitness nutrition for special dietary needs* (Champaign, IL: Human Kinetics). Reprinted, by permission, from E. Tribole, 2003, *Eating on the run,* 3rd ed. (Champaign, IL: Human Kinetics), 25.

Table 2.1 Nutrition Facts Label

Nutrition fact	Desirability	Comment
Calories	Not too many per serving	Be sure to check the serving size per package
Total fat	The lower, the better	Maximum 65 g per day
Saturated fat	The lower, the better	Maximum 20 g per day
Cholesterol	The lower, the better	Maximum 300 mg per day
Protein	Generally desirable	The average person needs only 54 g per day
Carbohydrate	Unless you are diabetic, not a key number to worry about	One average slice of bread has 15 g
Fiber	More is better	The average person gets only half of what he or she needs daily; aim for at least 25 g per day
Sugars	Less is better	4 g is equivalent to 1 tsp of sugar
Sodium	Less is better	Maximum 2,400 mg per day

Fiber

Fiber is a crucial component of the diet at any age, but it is particularly important for older adults. Although fiber is an indigestible carbohydrate, increasing dietary fiber provides many benefits, including

- lower blood lipid concentration,
- stable blood glucose concentration,
- decreased risk of coronary heart disease, and
- increased stool volume and promotion of a laxative effect, thus decreasing the risk of constipation and diverticulitis.

Both soluble and insoluble fiber are important. Soluble fiber is found in fruits, some legumes, and grains such as oats, rye, and barley. When consumed, soluble fiber forms a gel inside the digestive tract to slow the rate at which food passes through the small intestine. Subsequently, the rate of nutrient absorption increases, which is particularly important for older adults who may not be eating the variety of foods to which they were accustomed. Soluble fiber is also known for its benefit in lowering lipid concentration in the blood, namely total cholesterol levels.

Insoluble fiber is found primarily in vegetables and wheat bran. Insoluble fiber is important because it increases stool bulk. An easy way to increase fiber intake is through regular consumption of whole-grain cereals for breakfast: oatmeal, Shredded Wheat, bran flakes, and raisin bran are all good examples. Currently, the intake of dietary fiber in the United States is less than half the recommended values, which are 21 and 30 g of fiber per day, for females and males respectively.

Fat

Coronary heart disease is the number one killer of older adults in the United States. Although dietary fat is far from the only factor related to cardiovascular disease, epidemiological studies have shown a correlation between certain types of fat, like saturated and trans fat, and cardiovascular disease. Both saturated and trans fat may increase blood cholesterol concentrations as well as low-density lipoprotein cholesterol (LDL-C) concentrations in the blood. LDL-C is known as the bad cholesterol because it has the greatest effect on atherosclerosis. Trans fat is

produced during the hydrogenation of fat by food companies. These companies hydrogenate fat to increase the shelf life of certain foods and to give the fat a mouth feel closer to that of butter. Hydrogenation is also less expensive than using butter or another type of saturated fat. Hydrogenation changes the fat from its normal *cis* configuration to a *trans* configuration, which has negative effects on blood lipid concentration.

To minimize the negative effects of dietary fat, particularly its role in cardiovascular disease, people should consume no more than 20% to 35% of total energy from fat. A considerable body of evidence indicates that replacing saturated fat in the diet with monounsaturated and ***polyunsaturated fat***, particularly the omega-3 fats, has a positive effect on total ***blood lipid levels***. Therefore, of the total fat intake, about 13% should be derived from monounsaturated fat, about 10% should be derived from polyunsaturated fat, and less than 10% should be derived from saturated fat sources. Trans fat should also be kept to a minimum; these fats are found in many processed foods and other prepackaged food items. In the United States, all food labels provide the amount of trans fats in the product. At the time this book was written, only the United States had a requirement, which was fairly recent, to place the amount of trans fat on food labels. Australia, Canada, and countries in the European Union may require a similar disclosure in the near future. Table 2.2 summarizes major sources of fat and the effects of consuming different types of fat.

Vitamins and Minerals

Although overall energy needs decrease with age, the requirements for certain vitamins and minerals increase (table 2.3). In a publication in the *Journal of the American Medical Association*, Fletcher and Fairfield (2002) stated, "Pending strong evidence of effectiveness from randomized trials, it appears prudent for all adults to take vitamin supplements." Several nutrients are of particular concern (Blumberg, 1997). Although no supplement by itself can make up for a dietary deficiency, older adults should consider their need for particular nutrients.

A critical risk factor of malnutrition among older adults is their declining need for energy due to a reduction in lean body mass and lower activity levels. Vitamin deficiencies may not

Table 2.2 Sources and Health Effects of Fats

Fat type	Major sources	Effect on body
Monounsaturated fat	Olive oil, avocados, peanut butter, canola oil, hazel nuts, almonds, Brazil nuts, cashews, sesame seeds, pumpkin seeds, flaxseeds, and oil	Has been shown to decrease blood total cholesterol and LDL-C concentrations and may increase blood HDL-C concentrations
Polyunsaturated fat	Soybean oil, safflower oil, sunflower oil, corn oil, cottonseed oil, walnuts	Has been shown to decrease blood total cholesterol and LDL-C concentrations but may also slightly decrease HDL-C concentrations
Omega-3 fatty acids (long-chain polyunsaturated fatty acids)	Fatty fish (e.g., salmon, sardines, mackerel, herring, rainbow trout), canola oil, flaxseeds and oil, walnuts	Have been shown to decrease blood total cholesterol, LDL-C, and triglyceride concentrations
Saturated fat	Animal fats (butter, lard), fat in whole-fat dairy products	Has been shown to increase blood total cholesterol and LDL-C concentrations and lower HDL-C concentrations
Trans fat	Found in processed foods	Has been shown to increase blood total cholesterol and LDL-C concentrations and lower HDL-C concentrations

From S.L. Volpe, S. B. Sabelawski, and C.R. Mohr, 2007, *Fitness nutrition for special dietary needs* (Champaign, IL: Human Kinetics).

Table 2.3 Nutrient Needs of Older Adults for Selected Vitamins and Minerals

Nutrient	DRI for men (per day) 70 years of age or older	DRI for women (per day) 70 years of age or older	Food sources
Vitamin D (AI)	600 IU	600 IU	Fish liver oils, fatty fish, fortified milk and eggs
Calcium (AI)	1,200 mg	1,200 mg	Milk, cheese, yogurt, fortified tofu, fortified orange juice, greens, broccoli
Vitamin B$_{12}$ (RDA)	2.4 mg	2.4 mg	Fortified cereals, meat, fish, poultry
Vitamin B$_6$ (RDA)	1.7 mg	1.5 mg	Fortified grains, organ meats
Folate (RDA)	400 mcg	400 mcg	Enriched grains, dark leafy green vegetables, fortified cereals
Zinc (RDA)	11 mg	8 mg	Meats, seafood, fortified grains
Water (AI)	3.7 L/day	2.7 L/day	All beverages and high-moisture foods (e.g., watermelon, lettuce)[1]

AI = Adequate Intake; DRI = Dietary Reference Intake; IU = International Units; mg = milligram; mcg = microgram; L = liter; RDA = Recommended Daily Allowance

[1]Note that the recommendations for water are based on food and fluid intake; food provides about 20% of water needs, and fluids provide about 80% of water needs. Thus the DRI for water required per day does not mean that a person needs to consume that much plain water per day.

From S.L. Volpe, S.B. Sabelawski, and C.R. Mohr, 2007, *Fitness nutrition for special dietary needs* (Champaign, IL: Human Kinetics). Data from the Institute of Medicine Panel on Dietary Reference Intakes for Electrolytes and Water, 2004; Institute of Medicine Panel on Micronutrients, 2002; Institute of Medicine Standing Committee on the Scientific Evaluation of Dietary Reference Intakes, 1997; Institute of Medicine Panel on Folate, Other B Vitamins, and Chlorine and Institute of Medicine Subcommittee on Upper Reference Levels of Nutrients, 1998.

be detectable without actual biochemical and physical assessment, but any illness or stress, a common occurrence in older adults, may exacerbate subclinical deficiencies. Medications often interfere with vitamin absorption and usage (table 2.4). These interactions between medications and foods indicate the need for older adults to consume a nutrient-dense, well-balanced diet, full of variety. In addition, older adults should consult with their physicians, pharmacists, and registered dietitians for information regarding particular medications and their respective nutrient–medication interactions.

The vitamins and minerals that are most commonly deficient among the aging population are folate, calcium, zinc, and vitamins D, B_{12}, and B_6. Keep in mind that clinical malnutrition is not always apparent and is relatively uncommon in an otherwise healthy older population. Subclinical deficiencies, however, could lead to a number of health concerns, such as impaired immune function, impaired wound healing, muscle weakness, and fatigue, all of which would affect the day-to-day activities that are recommended for optimal health. The information that follows will help educate clients about how to avoid the most common vitamin and mineral deficiencies.

- **Vitamin D**. Vitamin D is a fat-soluble vitamin that, along with calcium, is crucial for bone health.

Table 2.4 Common Nutrient—Medication Interactions

Medication	Food	Interaction
Calcium channel blockers	Grapefruit and grapefruit juice	Grapefruit juice inhibits the enzymes needed to regulate the blood levels of these medications.
Coumadin	Foods high in vitamin K, such as green leafy vegetables, brussels sprouts, liver	Vitamin K in foods or supplements may reduce the effectiveness of the medication. Alcohol can increase the blood thinning effects of Coumadin.
Dilantin	Alcohol	Alcohol affects the way the body regulates Dilantin.
HMG-CoA reductase inhibitors (statins): Lipitor (Atorvastatin), Mevacor (Lovastatin), Zocor (Simvastatin)	Grapefruit and grapefruit juice	Grapefruit juice inhibits the enzymes needed to regulate the blood levels of these medications.
Lithium	Salt and caffeine	Lowering usual intake of salt and caffeine may cause lithium levels to rise, and increasing intake may have the opposite effect.
Monoamineoxidase inhibitors (MAOIs)	Foods high in tyramine, such as fermented, aged, or spoiled foods; aged cheeses; dry cured sausage meats; sauerkraut; yogurt; beer; red wine; soy sauce	Cause an increase in tyramine levels, leading to severe and potentially fatal hypertension.
Tetracycline	Calcium supplements or food sources of calcium	Calcium or calcium-rich foods reduce the absorption of tetracycline and should be avoided within 2 hours of taking the medication.

Note: This table is a guide for common medications. Individuals taking these medications should consult a physician, pharmacist, or registered dietitian for further information.

From S.L. Volpe, S.B. Sabelawski, and C.R. Mohr, 2007, *Fitness nutrition for special dietary needs* (Champaign, IL: Human Kinetics). Data from *Food Medication Interactions Handbook* (Pronsky, 2004).

Vitamin D intake and status have been shown to be low in older adults, with approximately 15% of the population deficient in the vitamin. This shortfall could result from a number of factors, such as decreased exposure to sunlight, which converts dietary vitamin D to its active form, and decreased milk consumption, a good source of vitamin D. Many older adults may not be exposed to the sun for the recommended 15 minutes per day for vitamin D conversion on the skin. Some may be homebound, and others may be covering up to protect themselves from skin cancer. Although this is a sound practice, older adults need to be educated that some sunlight every day (15 minutes per day) is needed to provide vitamin D. Milk is fortified with vitamin D, but because of taste preferences or lactose intolerance, which can develop with age, older adults often eliminate vitamin D from their diets. Vitamin D deficiency is common among homebound older adults; a negative correlation has been found between vitamin D and osteoporotic fractures. Of course, regular physical activity helps strengthen bones as well, but it cannot totally compensate for a deficient diet. Supplemental vitamin D of 400 International Units (IU) twice per day should be considered and is often included in comprehensive calcium supplements.

- **Calcium**. Calcium also plays an important role in the prevention of osteoporosis and helps maintain strong teeth. For men and women, the Dietary Reference Intake (DRI), established as an Adequate Intake (AI), for calcium increases at age 50 to 1,200 mg per day (Food and Nutrition Board [FNB], 1997). Ideally, calcium would all be derived from the diet; foods such as milk, cheese, yogurt, deep leafy green vegetables, broccoli, sardines, canned salmon with bones, dried beans and peas, tofu, and other calcium-fortified foods are great sources. Because many older adults no longer drink milk because of lactose intolerance, trying to convince them to consume lactose-free dairy products would be of benefit. Because 1,200 mg of calcium per day can be difficult for an older person to obtain through an energy-reduced diet, calcium supplements are often recommended. Calcium supplements come in several forms: carbonate, citrate, citrate malate, and so on. Refer to table 3.3 (page 45) to view the *bioavailability* of different forms of calcium supplementation. Calcium citrate (or calcium citrate malate) is often recommended because it does not need stomach acid for absorption, as calcium carbonate does. Because people produce less stomach acid as they age, supplementing with a form of calcium that does not require stomach acid for absorption is suggested. Depending on overall dietary intake, supplementing with 500 to 1,000 mg per day may be warranted.

- **Vitamin B_{12}, vitamin B_6, and folate**. Vitamin B_{12} is another common concern among older adults (Joosten et al., 1993). Inadequate absorption of the vitamin rather than inadequate dietary intake is responsible for more than 95% of the vitamin B_{12} deficiency seen in the United States. The usual cause of B_{12} deficiency is a loss of gastric intrinsic factor that is needed for absorption after the B_{12} is released from foods. The loss of intrinsic factor reduces the ability of the body to absorb vitamin B_{12}. Lack of proper absorption, or deficiency, of this vitamin typically results in elevated *homocysteine* levels or *megaloblastic anemia*. Folate supplementation can correct both conditions, but clinical work is necessary to determine the exact cause of the anemia or elevated homocysteine; otherwise, there is a possibility of masking one deficiency by increasing the dose of another vitamin. Moreover, some have suggested that folate and vitamin B_6 are also common deficiencies in the United States (Joosten et al.). Each of the three vitamins under discussion plays an important role in the reduction of homocysteine levels, which has been linked to cardiovascular disease. The best way to boost the intake of these B vitamins is to increase consumption of whole grains, which are often fortified with folate and are naturally high in the B vitamins.

- **Zinc**. Zinc intake is typically a function of overall energy intake; therefore, as energy intake declines, so does zinc consumption. As discussed, a decrease in energy intake is common among older adults. Zinc, a crucial component of over 300 metabolic reactions in the body, is important for immune health, hormone production, taste acuity, and wound healing. Therefore, nutritionists should recommend foods high in zinc (animal meats, fortified cereals, and certain seafood) and monitor the client's intake. The current RDA for zinc is 11 mg per day for men and 8 mg per day for women over 50 years of age.

Megaloblastic Anemia

Megaloblastic, or pernicious, anemia is a disorder in which the body does not absorb enough vitamin B_{12} from the digestive tract, resulting in decreased production of red blood cells. The decreased vitamin B_{12} absorption is often a result of an age-related decrease in the production of intrinsic factor, a substance that is found in stomach secretions and that is necessary for the absorption of vitamin B_{12}. Of note, megaloblastic anemia is more common in people of northern European descent than it is in any other ethnic group. Aside from aging, the inability of the body to synthesize intrinsic factor can also be a result of a gastrectomy, type 1 diabetes mellitus, thyroid disease, or having a family history of megaloblastic anemia.

Some signs and symptoms of megaloblastic (pernicious) anemia include muscle weakness, numbness or tingling in hands or feet, nausea, weight loss, decreased appetite, and diarrhea. People with megaloblastic anemia are often given a vitamin B_{12} injection on a monthly basis, but this therapy depends on the individual and the cause of the anemia.

Foods high in folate and vitamin B_{12} include eggs, meat, poultry, whole grains, milk, and shellfish.

Adapted from www.umm.edu/blood/aneper.htm.

Fluids

Generally, water receives little attention with regard to nutrient deficiencies. But water is by far the most important nutrient, serving a number of essential functions. Moreover, approximately one million elderly men and women are admitted to hospitals each year because of dehydration (Sansevero, 1997). A body-weight loss of as little as 1% results in impaired physiological and performance responses, demonstrating the importance of water. At the bottom of the Tufts Food Guide Pyramid for Older Adults (figure 2.1) is water, the foundation. Older adults should consume at least 8 cups (2 L) of water per day according to the pyramid. Dietary Reference Intakes for water have been established as an AI of 2.7 L per day for women and 3.7 L per day for men (FNB, 2004). Note that these recommendations do not imply that a person needs to drink 11 to 15 cups of straight water per day; a person can obtain the necessary water requirements from foods (on average, foods provide about 20% of water needs) and other fluids aside from pure water (for example, milk, 100% fruit juice, and coffee). Fluids provide 80% of water needs. Still, obtaining some of the water needs each day from water itself is important, because water does not provide excess energy. A good rule of thumb would be to obtain about three to four glasses per day from water itself if a person is also obtaining water from other fluids.

Adequate fluid intake reduces stress on kidney function, which often declines with age. In addition, adequate fluid intake eases constipation. A major issue is decreased ability to detect thirst, which declines with age, so encouraging fluid intake or providing some flavor to drinks to increase palatability is recommended. Regular physical activity increases fluid loss through sweating and thus requires water intake above DRI levels, so stressing the importance of water is crucial when making physical activity recommendations.

Dietary Supplements

Many vitamins and minerals act as *antioxidants* as part of the normal physiological functions in the body. An in-depth review of all antioxidants is beyond the scope of this chapter, but we present a basic overview here. Refer to the Web site http://nccam.nih.gov/ for information on approved claims for dietary supplements.

An often suggested method (particularly in advertising) of slowing the aging process is by taking dietary supplements, which are purported to do everything from helping to fight free radicals and enhancing cellular function to warding off or reducing the symptoms of disease. Although there are strong indications that various vitamins, minerals, and other nutrients are important in preventing some diseases or conditions, no consistently solid evidence supports a statement that supplementing with nutrient X or Z will provide a magic bullet against aging. For example, studies that have people take increased doses of vitamin E (about 400 IU per day) to help with Alzheimer's disease have not all shown positive benefits from this supplementation. Similarly, some people suggest that because various carotenoids, namely lutein and zeaxanthin,

Sample Meal Plan for Older Adults

Each meal plan provided is to be used as a guideline. Tables A.1 through A.4 in the appendix provide alternative food choices. We hope that this meal plan will provide a guide for foods from other countries that are similar in energy and nutrient content.

Breakfast

- 1 cup of bran flakes (fortified with iron and zinc) = 60 g
- 1 cup of low-fat milk = 240 ml
- 1/2 cup of strawberries = 20 g
- 1 slice toast = 40 g
- 1 tsp of margarine or butter = 5 g
- 8 oz of orange juice = 240 ml

Snack

- 1 cup of low-fat yogurt = 220 g
- 3 graham crackers (1 square each) = 10 g
- 1 medium pear = 100 g

Lunch

- 1 cup of split-pea soup or minestrone soup with lentils or beans = 240 ml
- 1 whole-wheat roll = 80 g
- 1 medium orange = 120 g
- 1 tsp of margarine or butter = 5 g

Snack

- 4 oz of vegetable or low-sodium vegetable juice = 120 ml
- 6 small whole-wheat cracker squares = 80 g
- 1 medium peach = 80 g

Dinner

- 4 oz of salmon (baked in 1/4 cup, or 20 g, of peach or regular salsa) = 120 g
- 1 cup of brown rice = 80 g
- 1 cup of steamed broccoli or asparagus = 60 g
- 1 whole-wheat dinner roll = 80 g
- 1 tsp of margarine or butter = 5 g
- 4 oz of low-fat frozen yogurt = 110 g

Snack

- 3 cups of light microwave popcorn = 90 g

This sample meal plan provides at least 100% of the Dietary Reference Intakes (DRIs) for energy, protein, fiber, vitamins A, C, E, B_6, B_{12}, thiamin, riboflavin, niacin, folate, calcium, iron, magnesium, phosphorus, zinc, and approximately

- 2,300 kcal (9,614 kJ),
- 100 g of protein,
- 50 g of fat,
- 33 g of fiber, and
- 4,200 mg of sodium.

From S.L. Volpe, S.B. Sabelawski, and C.R. Mohr, 2007, *Fitness nutrition for special dietary needs* (Champaign, IL: Human Kinetics).

are important to eye health, supplementing with increased doses above the amounts normally obtained in the diet will help. Again, making such recommendations without conclusive evidence is premature. Eating a variety of fruits, vegetables, whole grains, lean proteins, and healthy fats will provide many more nutrients than any single pill can provide. A maintenance-level multivitamin and mineral product has been recommended for all adults (Fletcher & Fairfield, 2002), but currently we have no clear evidence that older adults should supplement more with certain vitamins or minerals. Nonetheless, nutrition should be individualized, and if an older person requires specific nutrients, he or she should consult a registered dietitian.

A good rule to ensure adequate intake of vitamins, minerals, and antioxidants would be to consume at least two servings of dark leafy green vegetables per day and at least two servings of dark purple, red, or orange fruits or vegetables per day. These foods provide high levels of antioxidants that can help stave off cancer and cardiovascular disease, and possibly maintain eye health. Eating a cup of mixed berries (blueberries, strawberries, raspberries, or blackberries) each day is an excellent way to take in antioxidants.

PHYSICAL ACTIVITY

The importance of regular physical activity cannot be overestimated in the older population. People commonly accept that with aging comes a decline in muscle strength and elasticity, *insulin* sensitivity, bone strength, and ability to participate in activities of daily living (ADLs), such as walking up and down stairs, moving freely around the environment, getting in and out of chairs or the shower, and so forth. Fortunately, these negative factors are not associated as much with aging as they are with inactivity. A steep drop in strength and aerobic capacity is not inevitable; regular strength training and aerobic training can greatly slow the decline (Evans, 1999; Meredith, Zackin, Frontera, & Evans, 1987). Moreover, a meta-analysis conducted by Bonaiuti et al. (2002) concluded that aerobic, weight-bearing, and resistance exercises are all effective in increasing the bone mineral density of the spine in postmenopausal women, providing further evidence of the importance of regular activity. Granted, building bone

strength is optimized during youth, but the fact that the typical decreases are not necessary, and can be reduced, is important.

Benefits of Exercise for Older Adults

The benefits of exercise and physical activity have been well proved. People who exercise or are physically active on a daily basis have less risk of chronic disease, increased cognitive function, and greater ability to perform activities of daily living. Furthermore, exercise begun at any age can provide positive results.

Aerobic Exercise

Some have suggested that physical inactivity contributes as much to the risk of cardiovascular disease as smoking a pack of cigarettes each day! Cardiovascular function decreases 5% to 15% per decade after age 25 (Heath, Hagberg, Ehsani, & Holloszy, 1981), and maximal heart rate decreases an average of 6 to 10 beats per minute every decade (Fleg et al., 1995). The heart pumps blood less efficiently in older adults, and without regular physical activity to maintain its strength and integrity, the heart becomes even less efficient. Poor heart conditioning allows fatty and connective tissue to permeate the wall of the heart, exacerbating the decline in function. Fortunately, this decline is not inevitable with aging. The condition of the heart in adults who remain physically active is very different from that in people who are inactive. Because cardiovascular disease is the number one killer of older adults, regular cardiovascular activity is extremely important.

Reduced lung function is also a common issue with age. The effects of aging on the lungs are comparable to those that occur during the progression of mild emphysema. After about age 20, the number of alveoli and lung capillaries slowly begins to decrease, and by age 30, airway size and the number and elasticity of elastic fibers decrease. At about age 55, respiratory muscles start to weaken, and the chest wall slowly becomes less elastic. These effects are more profound in those who smoke or those who have had other environmental damage to their lungs (www.merck.com/mrkshared/mmg/sec10/ch75/ch75a.jsp). Although some of these changes are unavoidable, people who participate in regular aerobic exercise (walking, swimming, biking, jogging, and so forth) lessen some of the dramatic changes in pulmonary health and may be able to decrease the normal rate of loss that is common among aging people.

Older adults experience a decrease in insulin sensitivity. Researchers have shown, however, that regular physical activity improves insulin sensitivity, independent of weight loss (Hughes et al., 1995). Moreover, regular aerobic exercise may prevent the occurrence of type 2 diabetes mellitus, which is common among the older population. Furthermore, although some individuals can reduce hypertension by limiting salt intake, light- to moderate-intensity cardiovascular exercise also appears to lower blood pressure and improve lipid profiles. We have long known that aerobic exercise improves ***body composition*** by lowering body fat, even if overall body weight stays the same. Maintenance of lean body mass will also lead to greater ability to perform activities of daily living.

These benefits are the main health outcomes from participating in regular physical activity. Another important consideration is simply having a higher overall quality of life. Being able to play with grandchildren, walk without getting out of breath, and feel balanced and stable when moving all make life more enjoyable. Any type of cardiovascular exercise will suffice; the best exercise is one that the person enjoys enough to continue doing. Biking, swimming, walking, aerobic dance, or any form of exercise that elevates the heart rate continuously is fine. As long as it is performed on most, or preferably all, days of the week, tremendous health benefits will result.

Resistance Training

Aerobic exercise is the traditional exercise modality for those who are unaccustomed to regular activity, but resistance training is just as important, if not more important, in an overall fitness regimen for older adults (although any type of regular physical activity or movement can have

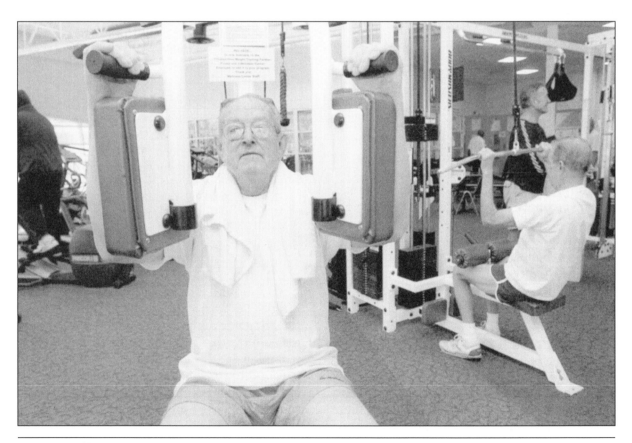

A regimen of basic strength exercises for your older clients will significantly increase their chances of remaining active for the majority of their remaining years.

a place in an overall fitness regimen). Research studies have shown dramatic increases in overall strength gains with the initiation of a resistance-training protocol. One study conducted on frail nursing-home residents (72 to 98 years of age) demonstrated significant gains in muscle strength and size, gait speed, stair-climbing power, and balance with a progressive resistance-training program. Moreover, in this study, spontaneous activity increased in the exercising group compared with the nonexercising group (Fiatarone et al., 1994). This study lends strong support to adding resistance exercise to the exercise protocols suggested to clients.

Besides improving muscle mass, resistance training can improve glucose tolerance, bone mineral density, strength, and balance, and decrease the risk of fractures. A person who is strong and maintains sufficient muscle mass will be more likely and able to perform regular aerobic exercises such as swimming, biking, or walking that require not only cardiovascular strength but also muscle strength. Increased muscular strength will allow older adults to rely on themselves to perform activities of daily living. This benefit alone is an important enhancement to the quality of life.

Balance and Flexibility Training

As people age, their overall balance decreases. Flexibility can decrease as well, but it can be maintained by daily performance of flexibility exercises. Maintaining balance and strength can lead to prevention of falls, which in turn prevents hip fractures, one of the most debilitating fractures for older adults. Simple exercises, such as standing on one leg while balancing oneself with the opposite hand on a stable chair or performing leg stretches while sitting in a chair or before rising out of bed each morning, are effective. Balance and flexibility exercises can be creative, performed almost anywhere, and can be performed several times throughout the day.

Exercise Prescription Guidelines for Older Adults

Clearly, then, exercise offers tremendous health advantages to older people. At the same time, however, exercise can be counterproductive if performed without observing proper safety guidelines. Older adults who exercise should follow several guidelines.

Myths About Older Adults and Resistance Training

Many people believe that older adults should avoid resistance training because they may injure themselves. But the opposite is true! Properly performed resistance training is crucial for older adults for many reasons. Many older adults (especially those older than age 80) are too weak to get out of a chair, prevent themselves from falling, or engage in simple activities of daily living. Resistance training has been shown to increase strength dramatically. When combined with a cardiovascular routine, resistance training will not only improve overall health but also may help prevent falls, improve mobility, and decrease the need for assistance with simple activities of daily living. The American College of Sports Medicine recommends that older adults perform

- at least one set of each of 8 to 10 exercises using major muscle groups,
- sets that involve 10 to 15 repetitions rated as somewhat hard on perceived exertion scales, and
- at least two training sessions per week, separated by at least 48 hours.

Older adults should consult a qualified exercise physiologist to ascertain whether they have any physical limitations or other situations, such as hypertension or diabetes mellitus, that may require special attention. Although the case study in this chapter is more complicated than most, the guest dietitian still included exercise as part of the overall plan for the patient.

• **Older adults should seek professional input.** The American College of Sports Medicine recommends a physician-supervised stress test for men over age 40 and for women over age 50 who plan to begin a vigorous exercise program (beyond basic walking or light resistance training) to ensure that no underlying signs or symptoms of disease would preclude participation. You should also recommend that your client seek the advice of a qualified person who can provide a suitable exercise prescription and instruction on technique and use of equipment.

- **Warming up and cooling down are important for older adults**. Like all adult exercisers, older adults should warm up before engaging in any physical activity. Slow treadmill walking or light cycling for 5 to 10 minutes is sufficient to achieve a slow increase in heart rate and circulation of blood throughout the body. Muscles need to be warm and pliable to reduce the risk of injury. Cooling down is also important. Sudden cessation of exercise can lead to venous pooling or lightheadedness. After completing an activity, a person should continue the same activity at lower intensity or simply walk for 3 to 5 minutes postexercise, before performing flexibility or stretching exercises.

- **Older exercisers should stretch appropriately**. Stretching is a crucial component of any exercise program. Older exercisers should seek the assistance of a qualified person to prescribe stretches for the large-muscle groups of the body. To reduce the risk of injury, stretches should be performed at the end of exercise sessions when blood flow is greater. Remember that muscles normally lose elasticity with aging. Without stretching, flexibility decreases, which can lead to injury and decrease the ability to perform activities of daily living.

- **Older adults should follow these guidelines for aerobic exercise**:
  - Older adults should engage in exercise that is comfortable and does not cause pain or discomfort.
  - They should perform at least 30 minutes of moderately intense physical activity on most, or preferably all, days of the week. Greater health benefits occur with higher doses of exercise; the more days per week that a person exercises, the more benefit he or she receives.

- **Older adults should follow these guidelines for resistance training**:
  - The exerciser should inhale before a lift and exhale during the exertion phase of the lift.
  - When pushing against resistance, the exerciser should avoid rapid breathing or hyperventilating.
  - Isometric and static resistance exercises are not recommended.
  - The older adult should work with a qualified trainer who can periodically measure

blood pressure response during the workout.
  - Resistance used can be anything that is above and beyond normal movement (for example, soup cans placed inside an old purse can be the weight used for biceps and triceps curls, leg lifts, and leg curls).
  - Exercises should focus on large-muscle groups. The bench press, leg press, and squats are good choices. A qualified trainer should assist with developing proper form.
  - The weight used should put a comfortable strain on the muscles being used to perform the movement.

CASE STUDY

Joseph was a 75-year-old African American male. He weighed 94.2 lb (43 kg), which is 52% of his ideal body weight.

He lived with a roommate and had an extensive medical history of type 2 diabetes, diabetic nephropathy, and cataracts.

A biochemical evaluation revealed chronic **hypoalbunemia**, which may have been a result of chronic malnutrition. His **glycosylated hemoglobin** levels strongly suggest uncontrolled diabetes as a result of infection, poor diet, and chronic malnutrition. All other biochemical labs were within baseline. A clinical observation also revealed the patient had **cachexia** with marked muscle wasting. Our goal was to bring him to a healthy body weight, while we monitored his diabetes mellitus and other comorbidities.

Joseph admitted to having a poor appetite and poor intake for the past 2 to 3 years following several surgeries. His body weight was 150 lb (68.1 kg) 2 to 3 years ago. The patient stated that he does not cook for himself. He lives with a friend, but she has difficulty ambulating and cooking. Joseph states that Meals on Wheels would make his life and his roommate's life much easier.

Present Medications

The client currently takes Megace, Creon, Simvastatin, NPH insulin, vitamin B_{12}, and iron sulfate.

It is important for him to take Creon with meals because it helps digestion in certain conditions when the pancreas is not working properly. If the pancreas is unable to produce the enzymes that digest starch, fat, and protein, Creon is used. Creon contains the pancreatic enzymes needed for digestion of proteins, starches, and fats.

Estimation of Protein and Energy Requirements

The first step in estimating the patient's energy requirement was to find his ideal weight. Given his height and adjusting for a small frame, his ideal weight would be 160 lb (72.7 kg). Multiplying that figure by 25 to 30 kcal per kg (105 to 125 kJ per kg) of body weight produced an estimated energy requirement of 1,800 to 2,200 kcal (7,524 to 9,196 kJ) per day.

The patient's protein requirement was estimated to be 85 g of protein per day, found by multiplying the patient's ideal body weight by 1.2 grams of protein per kg of body weight. (To convert body weight in pounds to body weight in kilograms, take body weight in pounds and divide it by 2.2 to calculate body weight in kilograms.)

Summary and Plan

The patient has an infection on his left ankle and face. A workup revealed that he had cellulitis.

I recommended a 2,200 kcal per day (9,196 kJ per day) diabetic diet with 106 g of protein. I also suggested the use of Diabetic Resource fruit beverage or other diabetic nutritional supplement with his meals three times a day.

I also recommended that he meet with an exercise physiologist to begin a mild exercise routine within his current physical limitations. Walking is a simple activity that does not require skill, but the exercise physiologist will provide an appropriate exercise prescription (intensity, frequency, and duration) after he or she consults with the patient.

Goals

- Encourage the patient to maintain a diabetic diet of 2,200 kcal per day (9,196 kJ per day) with a nutritional supplement.
- Discuss the availability of Meals on Wheels.
- Monitor strategies for improved dietary intake.
- Weigh daily when tolerable.
- Continue monitoring blood glucose levels for glucose control.
- Monitor serum albumin and prealbumin levels for protein status.

Sarah Michelle Agena, MS, RD
Assistant Manager and Fitness Director
Miracles Fitness
West Lafayette, Indiana

Menopause

Many women will spend one-third of their lives past menopause.

Menopause is a time of drastic hormonal change for women. Many women must cope with hot flashes, weight gain, and mood swings, among many other undesirable side effects. Proper nutrition and exercise can play an important role in minimizing, and possibly preventing, some of these unpleasant physiological changes that occur surrounding menopause.

PHYSIOLOGICAL CHANGES IN MENOPAUSE

Menopause is defined as the absence of menstrual periods for 12 consecutive months. This time is also accompanied by lower levels of estrogen, which is the major female hormone. Estrogen has many functions besides maintaining the menstrual cycle, as detailed in "*Roles of Estrogen in the Body*." Menopause can also be defined as the time when follicular cells in the ovary do not produce **follicle stimulating hormone (FSH),** which causes the ovaries to cease producing viable eggs, which then leads to a decrease in estrogen and **progesterone** (Bass, 2001).

Roles of Estrogen in the Body

- Causes deposition of fat into the breasts
- Results in increased bone mineral density
- Increases protein and fat deposition
- Increases metabolism slightly
- Results in softer, smoother, and thicker skin than in children
- Affects electrolyte balance (sodium and water retention) slightly

Adapted from A.C. Guyton and J.E. Hall, 1996, *Textbook of medical physiology* (Philadelphia, PA: WB Saunders Co).

The average age of the onset of menopause is 51 years, but it can begin as early as age 30. Poor nutrition and smoking can result in earlier menopause; conversely, women who started their menstrual cycles later in life typically begin menopause later in life. A number of symptoms associated with menopause are listed in the section "*Symptoms Associated With Menopause.*"

Perimenopause is defined as changes in the menstrual cycle (for example changes in

Symptoms Associated With Menopause

- Hot flashes
- Night sweats
- Vaginal dryness
- Insomnia
- Urinary tract problems
- Poor concentration
- Dry hair and skin
- Mood swings
- Heart palpitations

- Irritability or anxiety
- Depression
- Headaches
- Memory loss
- Changes in sexual desire
- Joint pain

Adapted from D.G. von Muhlen, D. Kritz-Silverstein and E. Barrett-Conno, 1995, "A community-based study of menopause symptoms and estrogen replacement in older women," *Maturitas* 22(2): 71-78.

regularity) before menopause. Although *peri* means "around," perimenopause can occur as early as 10 years before the onset of menopause. During this time, estrogen levels start to decline.

Postmenopause occurs 5 years or longer after menopause, but the hormonal changes that accompany postmenopause occur several years before its actual onset (Bass, 2001). Symptoms of postmenopause include vaginal dryness and itchiness, high blood pressure, stress incontinence, bone fractures, skin wrinkles, hot flashes, sleep disturbances, irritability, fatigue, and decreased libido. Many of these symptoms are the same as those that occur in menopause, but after menopause is complete the symptoms tend to be less severe.

NUTRITION

Most readers are familiar with the most common signs and symptoms of menopause: hot flashes, mood swings, dry skin, coarsening of hair, vaginal dryness, and night sweats. But nutritional measures can minimize some long-term diseases commonly associated with menopause. The two most common and serious of these are osteoporosis and cardiovascular disease (CVD). Diet can have a positive effect on all these conditions—both general signs and symptoms as well as the long-term diseases. We will discuss the potential effect of diet on the general symptoms first and then consider osteoporosis and CVD. The section closes with an extensive table that summarizes the nutritional needs of both active and sedentary women in perimenopause, menopause, and postmenopause.

General Menopausal Symptoms

We have already described the general symptoms of menopause, so we will go right into consideration of dietary strategies to address them. Because phytoestrogens are an important element in the ideal diet for older women, we will devote a section to these compounds and will group other recommendations in their own segment. The section *"Minimizing Menopausal Symptoms Through Diet"* provides general strategies that your clients can use, whereas the following sections provide detail and specific recommendations. Table 3.5 (pages 50-53) summarizes nutrition recommendations for active menopausal women.

Consuming Phytoestrogens

Phytoestrogens have been a hot topic in the media and in the scientific literature for the past 10 years. What exactly are phytoestrogens? They are compounds that occur naturally in plant foods (vegetables and fruits) and have an estrogen-like action in the body. But they do not have the potency of the estrogen produced in the body. Nonetheless, phytoestrogens have been used clinically for the treatment of high blood cholesterol, menopausal symptoms, and cancer prevention. Note that phytoestrogens are not a cure, but they can be helpful. Because many people in the United States do not consume a large amount of fruits and vegetables on a daily basis, increased consumption of fruits and vegetables will naturally increase the consumption of phytoestrogens. Up to 94 foods contain phytoestrogens, but the content in each food varies (Lange-Collett, 2002).

Phytoestrogens fall into four main groups, as shown in table 3.1. Specific foods rich in phytoestrogens are listed by type in table 3.2. You may photocopy both tables for your clients.

The mechanism of action of phytoestrogens relates to their ability to bind with estrogen receptor sites (Lange-Collett, 2002). When high levels of circulating estrogen are available, relatively little binding occurs in the receptor sites. As the levels of estrogen decrease, however, the binding capacity of phytoestrogens increases to supplement the deficiencies in the body (Lange-Collett).

As estrogen levels decrease, the symptoms of perimenopause may arise. These symptoms

Minimizing Menopausal Symptoms Through Diet

Although not all symptoms of menopause are related to nutrition, nutrition recommendations can ease some of them. Note that these recommendations are not perfect and may help some women more than they help others. To minimize hot flashes, women should avoid stimulants like caffeine and alcohol as well as heat-producing foods such as spicy foods and hot beverages. Nausea can be minimized by decreasing the consumption of acidic foods (tomatoes and orange juice, for example), especially on an empty stomach. Reducing the intake of high-sugar foods and concentrated sweets, especially on an empty stomach, may help diminish mood swings because consumption of these foods can cause a rapid increase and then a decrease in blood sugar, which can be related to irritability. Headaches can be curtailed by decreasing the consumption of red wine, beer, coffee, and chocolate. Alcohol and caffeine are frequent triggers for headaches in some people (Bass, 2001).

From S.L. Volpe, S.B. Sabelawski, and C.R. Mohr, 2007, *Fitness nutrition for special dietary needs* (Champaign, IL: Human Kinetics).

Table 3.1 Four Main Groups of Phytoestrogens and Their Food Sources

Phytoestrogen	Food sources
Isoflavone	Legumes (soybeans, lentils, barlotti, broad, haricot, lima beans, kidney beans), soy milk, soy flour, tofu, miso, soy cheese
Lignans	Cereals, fruits, vegetables, linseed and flaxseeds; smaller concentrations in whole-grain cereals (e.g., wheat, barley, oats, rye, brown rice, bran)
Coumestans	Similar to foods high in isoflavones
Resocyclic acid lactones (mycotoxins)	Produced by mold growing in damp conditions; not true phytoestrogens; usually removed in the preparation and refining of the product

From S.L. Volpe, S.B. Sabelawski, and C.R. Mohr, 2007, *Fitness nutrition for special dietary needs* (Champaign, IL: Human Kinetics).

Table 3.2 Foods Rich in Phytoestrogens

Soy products	Grains	Legumes	Vegetables	Fruits	Others
Soybeans	Wheat germ	Lentils	Alfalfa	Apples	Garlic
Soy flour	Barley	Black or red beans	Carrots	Pears	Olive oil
Tofu, miso, tempeh	Rye	Chickpeas	Fennel	Cherries	Tea (green or black)
Bean curd	Rice bran		Onions	Stone fruits	Hops
Soy milk	Oat bran		Corn		Some seeds and nuts

From S.L. Volpe, S.B. Sabelawski, and C.R. Mohr, 2007, *Fitness nutrition for special dietary needs* (Champaign, IL: Human Kinetics).

include drying of the skin, coarser hair, decreased vaginal lubrication, and decreased bone mass. Replacing the declining estrogen levels may reduce these symptoms. Daily soy supplementation has been shown to decrease the frequency of hot flashes by 40% to 45%. Although phytoestrogen intake may not decrease hot flashes in all women, increased consumption of soy products may be a more natural approach for women who experience night sweats.

Natural phytoestrogens are not as potent as hormone replacement therapy (HRT) or estrogen replacement therapy (ERT). Nonetheless, although more research is required to establish the effects that soy products have on menopausal symptoms, increased soy consumption can still be beneficial for overall health. You can print out both *"Adding Phytoestrogens to Your Diet"* and table 3.2, "Foods Rich in Phytoestrogens" (page 43), for your older female clients to encourage them to increase phytoestrogens in their diets.

Other Nutritional Strategies

Consuming soy isoflavones and flaxseed may help alleviate general symptoms of menopause for some women. Neither is effective for everyone, and if a person has any questions, she should consult a registered dietitian or physician before trying anything new.

- **Soy**. Some studies have indicated that the *isoflavones* in soy, and isoflavones in general, can ease hot flashes, but other studies found only a slight reduction. Isoflavones are estrogen-like *phytochemicals* that produce estrogen-like activity in the body. Safe levels of isoflavones have not yet been established; therefore, many questions remain about how consumption of excess amounts of isoflavones may affect healthy women. According to Dr. Mark Messina (Bass, 2001), 15 g of soy protein and 50 mg of isoflavones are good levels to consume. Women should not consume more than 25 to 30 g per day of soy

Adding Phytoestrogens to Your Diet

These foods are good sources of phytoestrogens and should be included in the diet each day.

- Two to four slices of soy-enriched bread per day
- Two servings (8 oz, or 240 ml, each) of soy milk per day (calcium enriched if your calcium intake is low), consumed alone or with hot or cold cereals
- 1 tbsp (15 g) of flaxseed per day (add it to cereals or yogurt)
- One soy-based vegetarian burger (2 to 3 oz, or 60 to 90 g)
- Variety of legumes, whole grains and cereals, fruits, and vegetables
- Chickpeas added to salads
- Canned beans added to soups or salads
- Tofu or ground soy for meat casseroles
- Green soybeans as a substitute for peas or beans
- Soy cheese added to sandwiches

From S.L. Volpe, S.B. Sabelawski, and C.R. Mohr, 2007, *Fitness nutrition for special dietary needs* (Champaign, IL: Human Kinetics).

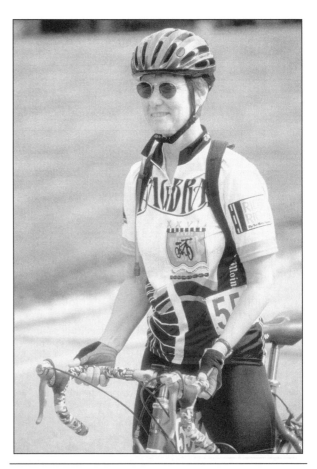

Following the best nutritional practices for menopause and postmenopause can optimize an older woman's chances of pursuing an active and enjoyable lifestyle.

protein and not more than 100 mg per day of isoflavones (100 mg of isoflavones are found in 10.5 oz, or 280 g, of tofu; in 3/4 cup, or 90 g, of shelled edamame (soy beans); or in 5 cups, or 1.2 L, of soy milk) (Bass). The bottom line is that increasing soy consumption in the diet will be beneficial, but a woman should not overdo the consumption, thinking that more is better.

• **Ground flaxseed**. Increased fluid intake must accompany increased flaxseed consumption (and increased fiber consumption overall), because consuming more fiber without increasing fluid consumption can cause constipation.

Common Diseases in Menopause

One of the main goals of nutrition professionals is to help clients make healthy choices to prevent chronic diseases such as osteoporosis and cardiovascular disease. These chronic diseases are commonly assumed part of the aging process. They do not have to be. As discussed in chapter 2, following a healthy diet and staying physically active can prevent or delay many of these diseases.

Osteoporosis

Osteoporosis is probably the most well-known disease that can occur after menopause because postmenopausal osteoporosis is directly related to the loss of estrogen that occurs rapidly during menopause. Because bone contains receptors for estrogen that increase bone mineral density (BMD), after the estrogen in the body decreases, BMD decreases as well. Note that bone loss usually stabilizes at about 75 years of age, but this is not true for all people, especially those who get "senile osteoporosis," which is typically associated with bone loss as we age. Although diet cannot prevent osteoporosis entirely, in many cases it can slow its progress. You should recommend the following nutritional measures to your clients who are approaching, already in, or past menopause.

• **Calcium**. During the first 5 years of menopause, calcium supplementation does not really help with bone loss because of the dramatic decrease in estrogen levels. Consuming 1,000 to 1,500 mg of calcium per day remains important, however, because the body still requires calcium, and even more of it as people age. This calcium intake translates to about four 8 oz (240 ml) glasses of milk per day (because an 8 oz glass of milk provides about 300 mg of calcium). Those who cannot tolerate milk can take 500 mg of a calcium supplement in the morning and the same dosage in the evening, with 200 International Units (IU) of vitamin D with each supplement, to help slow the progression of osteoporosis. By dividing the calcium into two doses, more of it will be absorbed. The best supplement is calcium citrate, because it has the highest percent absorption. Calcium from oyster shell or shark cartilage should be avoided because of the higher levels of mercury and lead in these types of supplements. See table 3.3 for a list of

Table 3.3 Comparison of Calcium Supplements to Milk

Form	Percent of recommended intake of calcium[1]	Percent calcium absorption from each supplement or milk	Amount of lead (mg) in each supplement or milk
Carbonate (500 mg of elemental calcium)	~40%	26%	0.92
Oyster shell (500 mg of elemental calcium)[2]	~30%	26%	~5 to 11
Citrate (500 mg of elemental calcium)	~21%	35%	1.64
Milk (8 oz, or 240 ml)	~30%	33%	0.71

[1]The Dietary Reference Intakes (DRI), established as Adequate Intakes (AI) for calcium are 1,000 mg/day for women 31 to 50 years of age and 1,200 mg/day for women >50 years of age (Food and Nutrition Board, 1997).

[2]Not recommended but listed to show high levels of lead contained in this type of supplement.

Adapted from D.I. Levenson, 1994.

calcium supplements compared with milk. Skim milk provides the same amount of calcium as whole or low-fat milk does, but it does not have saturated fat, which means that it is a healthier choice. Table 3.4, which you may photocopy for your clients, provides information on the calcium content of other dairy food sources.

• **Protein**. Another nutritional way that people can minimize bone loss is to avoid consuming too much protein. Protein is an important part of any diet, but research has shown that over-consumption of protein may cause higher loss of calcium in the urine. If that happens, less of that calcium will have been used to build up or maintain bone mass. The standard recommendation is that people consume about 0.8 g of protein per kg of body weight, or about 0.5 g protein per lb of body weight (Food and Nutrition Board [FNB], 1997). People should try not to consume more than twice this amount on a regular basis.

• **Caffeine**. Drinking 1 cup of coffee results in a loss of about 3.5 mg of calcium in the urine. The good news is that adding milk or half-and-half to coffee offsets the calcium loss. Those who drink a large amount of black coffee each day will lose a significant amount of calcium in the urine, and they may want to cut back on their coffee consumption. Those who find it too difficult to change their coffee-consuming habit should be sure to consume an amount of calcium at the upper end of the range (1,500 mg) each day. Other calcium robbers are caffeinated sodas, tea, and chocolate. Tea and chocolate offer wonderful benefits as antioxidants, but consuming too much of these products can result in more calcium loss because of the caffeine. So, people should be sure to consume a good balance of healthy foods.

• **Phosphorus**. Intakes of phosphorus can lead to bone loss if they are high enough to change the ratio of calcium to phosphorus from the recommended 2:1 or 1:1 to 1:2 or 1:3. Like other nutrients, phosphorus consumed within the recommended intakes (700 mg per day for adults) will help maintain good bone health, but overconsumption of this mineral can be harmful to bone and other functions in the body. Although

Table 3.4   Calcium and Phosphorus Content of Some Commonly Consumed Foods

Food	Calcium content (mg)	Phosphorus content (mg)
1/2 cup of macaroni	8	47
1/2 cup of artichokes	51	69
1/2 cup of broccoli	88	62
1/2 cup of collards	152	39
1/2 cup of swiss chard	184	37
1/2 cup of okra	92	41
1/2 cup of almonds	120	260
1 cup of baked beans	155	175
1/2 cup (120 ml) of chocolate milk	26	28
1 cup of milk (240 ml)	300	235
1 cup of yogurt	400	250
1 cup of cottage cheese	138	236
1 oz (28 g) of cheddar cheese	204	145
1 cup of kefir	300	200

Note: 1/2 dry cup = about 55 g; 1 dry cup = about 110 g; 1 liquid cup = 240 ml; 1/2 liquid cup = 120 ml; 1 oz = about 28 g.

From S.L. Volpe, S.B. Sabelawski, and C.R. Mohr, 2007, *Fitness nutrition for special dietary needs* (Champaign, IL: Human Kinetics). Adapted from P. Insel, R.E. Turner, and D. Ross, 2001, *Nutrition* (Boston, MA: Jones and Bartlett).

the tolerable upper limit for phosphorus is 4 g per day for adults, people should not strive to consume that much (FNB, 1997). Some significant dietary sources of phosphorus are listed in table 3.4. Consumption of these foods should be limited to avoid overconsumption of phosphorus.

- **Carbonated beverages**. Older women should avoid carbonated beverages. A soda now and then is not harmful, but drinking more than two sodas per week is not advisable. Sodas provide no nutritional benefit, and if consumed in any significant quantity, they are harmful to the health of older women. Many sodas contain caffeine and sugar, and all of them contain phosphorus. We have seen that both caffeine and phosphorus promote the leaching of calcium from the bones, an occurrence that no older woman can afford to experience. And sugared sodas are one of the main contributors to the obesity epidemic currently afflicting modern developed societies. Because extra weight puts added stress on bones that are osteoporotic or are approaching that condition, older women should do all they can to keep their weight at a healthy level, including cutting down on the number of sugar-containing carbonated beverages that they drink.

- **Soy protein**. Although the evidence is still inconclusive, soy protein may be protective of bone, especially if it is fortified with calcium. Soy contains *phytoestrogens* (plant estrogens), which can somewhat mimic the estrogen that the body produced before menopause. This can result in bone accretion, or buildup. But the amount of soy needed to result in the accretion of bone has not been fully established. A recently published study found that increased soy protein did not improve calcium retention in postmeno-

pausal women, suggesting that it may not be protective of bone (Spence et al., 2005). Others have also reported no effects of soy protein on bone density in either animals or humans (Arjmandi et al., 2005; Nakai, Black, Jefferey, & Barr, 2005), although some have reported improvements in markers of bone with 25 g per day of soy protein (Arjmandi et al.). More research is required in the area of bone metabolism and soy protein intake before we can make definitive statements. Nonetheless, soy protein is a great addition to the diet because it may help reduce the risk of cancer and cardiovascular disease.

- **High-fiber diets**. High-fiber diets may also lead to calcium loss because the phytates and *oxalates* in plant foods bind to minerals, thus decreasing their overall absorption. But fiber is a wonderful constituent of our diets, and it should be consumed at levels of about 25 to 35 g per day to promote regular bowel movements and help prevent colon cancer and cardiovascular disease. Again, people should be aware that too much of a good thing is not always good for them!

Cardiovascular Disease

Cardiovascular disease (CVD) is the leading cause of death among women, especially postmenopausal women. Over 50% of all women in the developed world will die of CVD (Lange-Collett, 2002).

The rate of CVD is especially high among postmenopausal women because after menopause, blood levels of low-density lipoprotein cholesterol (LDL-C) increase. LDL-C, known as the bad cholesterol, results in increased plaque formation within the arteries and vessels of our bodies. Research has shown that the following nutritional

Smoking and Bone Health Do Not Mix

If your female clients want strong bones, here are three good reasons that they should not smoke:

- Nicotine blocks estrogen receptors, which decreases bone accretion, resulting in bone *resorption,* or breakdown, that causes smokers to have lower average bone mineral density than nonsmokers do.
- Women smokers reach menopause up to 2 years earlier than nonsmokers do and thus are at greater risk of osteoporosis because they do not have the endogenous (made internally in the body) estrogens in their body for as long a time (North American Menopause Society, 2002).
- We know that smoking greatly increases the risks of lung cancer. The chemotherapy or radiation therapy that is a common treatment for cancer often results in early menopause.

strategies combat these effects of menopause or may be helpful in combating these effects. Remember that people respond differently (or not at all) to certain strategies.

• **Soy protein**. Studies of premenopausal women have indicated a significant reduction in CVD risk with long-term soy consumption (Lange-Collett, 2002). The exact amount of soy consumption has not been established, but an approved health claim states that 25 g of soy protein per day, as part of a diet low in saturated fat and cholesterol, may reduce the risk of heart disease. This benefit is most likely a result of the isoflavones (a form of antioxidants) within the soy that help to increase high-density lipoprotein cholesterol (HDL-C) in the blood and lower the levels of LDL-C. HDL-C, known as the good cholesterol, helps to get rid of the LDL-C and decrease plaque formation in the blood vessels.

• **Iron**. Monitoring the intake of iron after menopause is important. Excessive iron intake has been shown to increase CVD risk. In general, women who consume too much iron are usually supplementing their dietary intake with iron supplements. To avoid excessive iron intake, a woman should supplement with iron only if she has iron deficiency anemia and has been prescribed iron supplements by her physician. Recent research suggests that increased blood iron and copper levels, combined with decreased blood zinc and selenium concentrations, can also result in increased markers of CVD risk (Altekin et al., 2005).

• **C-reactive protein**. A fairly new measure for assessing the risk of heart disease is something called *C-reactive protein (CRP)*. This has been shown to be a better indicator of risk of heart disease than blood lipid levels alone. That is not to say that people should not be aware of their LDL-C, HDL-C, and total cholesterol levels, but they should pay attention to C-reactive protein levels as well. C-reactive protein is a plasma protein that measures acute inflammation. Recent evidence suggests that elevated levels of C-reactive protein may increase a person's risk for cardiovascular disease. Normal values of C-reactive protein are less than 0.6 mg per deciliter (dl) (www.nlm.nih.gov/medlineplus/ency/article/003356.htm).

• **Decreasing saturated fat**. Decreasing the amount of saturated fat in the diet will help decrease CVD risk, especially after menopause. Because a woman's risk of CVD increases after menopause, reducing saturated fat intake can be one step that she takes to help decrease her risk. Increased saturated fat intake (for example, animal fats such as butter, lard, and whole milk) leads to increases in serum total cholesterol and low-density lipoprotein cholesterol concentrations and reductions in high-density lipoprotein cholesterol concentrations. Refer to chapter 2, "Aging," for more information about fat intake.

• **Omega-3 fatty acids and flaxseeds**. *Omega-3 fatty acids* are long-chained, polyunsaturated fatty acids. Omega-3 fatty acids and flaxseeds, as well as flaxseed oil, are excellent sources of isoflavones. Omega-3 fatty acids are found mainly in fatty fish (for example, tuna, salmon, monkfish) and ground flaxseed (greater fiber content) or flaxseed oil. Although omega-3 fatty acids have been shown to decrease blood triglyceride levels and increase blood HDL-C levels, they also may increase blood concentrations of total cholesterol and LDL-C (Castro, Barroso, & Sinnecker, 2005; Putadechakum et al., 2005). Although

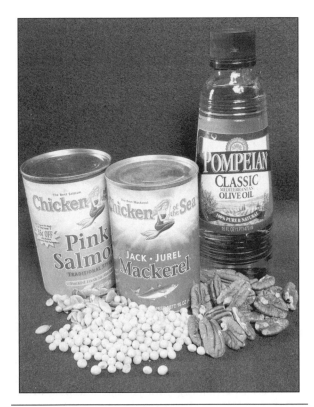

Consuming fatty fish twice a week, using olive oil as her main cooking and salad oil, and eating seeds or nuts daily can help a woman increase her HDLs and lower her overall cholesterol level.

Sample Meal Plan for Menopausal Women

This meal plan is intended for moderately active women and should be individualized as appropriate for specific needs. For example, a woman who is active but needs less energy would need to decrease the portion sizes to meet her individual needs. See tables A.1 through A.4 in the appendix for alternative food choices.

Breakfast

- 1 cup of bran or whole-grain flakes = 60 g
- 1 cup of skim milk or calcium-fortified low-fat soy milk = 240 ml
- 3/4 cup of blueberries = 35 g
- 8 oz of orange juice (calcium-fortified) = 240 ml
- 1 cup of coffee = 240 ml
- 1 tsp of half-and-half or skim milk for coffee = 5 ml
- 1 tsp of sugar or honey for coffee = 5 g

Snack

- 8 whole-wheat crackers = 80 g
- 2 tbsp of peanut butter = 30 g
- 1 medium apple = 80 g
- 8 oz of water = 240 ml

Lunch

- Tuna salad sandwich
  - -2 oz of tuna salad = 56 g
  - -2 slices of whole-grain bread = 80 g
  - -2 slices each of lettuce and tomato = 10 g
  - -1 tsp of mayonnaise = 5 g
  - -1 tsp of lemon juice = 5 ml
- 1 cup of vegetable soup = 240 ml
- 1 cup of skim milk or calcium-fortified low-fat soy milk = 240 ml

Snack

- 1 cup of low-fat yogurt = 220 g
- 6 vanilla wafers = 80 g
- 8 oz of water = 240 ml

Dinner

- Grilled chicken breast over salad
  - -2 oz of grilled chicken breast = 60 g
  - -2 cups of mixed greens salad = 60 g
  - -1/4 cup of grape tomatoes = 10 g
  - -2 tbsp of balsamic vinaigrette dressing = 28 g
- 1/2 cup of lentil soup = 120 ml
- 1/2 cup of skim milk or calcium-fortified low-fat soy milk = 120 ml

Snack

- 3 cups of light microwave popcorn = 90 g
- 8 to 12 oz of water = 240 to 360 ml

This sample meal plan provides at least 100% of the Dietary Reference Intakes (DRIs) for energy (kilocalories), protein, fiber, vitamins A, C, E, B_6, B_{12}, thiamin, riboflavin, niacin, folate, calcium, iron, magnesium, phosphorus, zinc, and approximately

- 2,300 kcal (9,614 kJ),
- 94 g of protein,
- 68 g of fat,
- 34 g of fiber, and
- 3,300 mg of sodium.

From S.L. Volpe, S.B. Sabelawski, and C.R. Mohr, 2007, *Fitness nutrition for special dietary needs* (Champaign, IL: Human Kinetics).

increased consumption of both omega-3 fatty acids and flaxseeds may be beneficial, being aware of the appropriate seasons to consume certain types of fish is important in minimizing mercury consumption. As always, the key is to consume a good balance of all types of foods and avoid focusing on certain foods (or supplements). Some of the health benefits of consuming omega-3 fatty acids are that they reduce inflammation, are antithrombotic (that is, they break up clots), and are nonimmunoreactive.

- **Garlic.** Garlic is often used as a supplement to help decrease CVD by possibly lowering serum total cholesterol concentrations and high blood pressure. In addition, garlic consumption has been shown to inhibit or prevent some types of cancers. Some people eat garlic cloves raw, but garlic can be beneficial in dried, powdered, or tablet or capsule form without having the unpleasant odor. People should be cautious when taking supplemental garlic because it tends to thin the blood and reduces the ability of the blood to clot. Therefore, anyone planning to have any type of surgical procedure should discontinue garlic supplementation for at least 1 week beforehand. As always, people should inform their health care providers about any types of supplements (dietary or herbal) that they are taking.

Table 3.5 summarizes nutritional recommendations for menopausal women, both those who exercise and those who do not. Note that these are general guidelines and that nutritional recommendations should be individualized. You may photocopy the table for your clients or patients.

Table 3.5 Nutrition for Active Menopausal and Postmenopausal Women

Nutrient	General recommendations	Recommendations for athletes	Food sources	Why do we need these?	Considerations
Energy (kcal or kJ)	2,403 kcal/day	≥2,403 kcal/day (10,045 kJ/day)	Most food sources (those that contain carbohydrate, fat, or protein)	Required to sustain life	Women who exercise more frequently, at higher intensities, may need more kilocalories than stated, and women who are less active will need slightly fewer kilocalories.
Carbohydrate (CHO)	130 g/day	300 to 500 g/day	Whole grains, pasta, fruits, rice, vegetables, breads, cereals	Ideal fuel to improve overall performance, supply the brain and body with power, and produce stores of glycogen	Choose whole grains and avoid refined carbohydrate and sweets.
Protein	0.4 g/lb (0.2 g/kg)	0.45 to 0.9 g/lb[1] (0.2 to 0.41 g/kg)	Lean meats, fish, poultry, shellfish, eggs, soy products, low-fat milk or dairy products, legumes, hummus	Maintains and repairs cells, produces enzymes and hormones, and supplies energy when not available from CHO	More than 0.9 g/lb (>0.41 g/kg) of protein • will not enhance muscle development, • can compromise CHO intake, which can decrease the ability to train at peak levels, • causes diuresis (increased urination), which may lead to dehydration, and • is stored as fat.
Fat[2]	≤30% of total energy (kcal or kJ) intake	0.45 g/lb (0.21 g/kg)		Provides essential fatty acids (EFAs), hormones, immunity, and fat-soluble vitamins, and is a good source of energy	
Water and fluids	64 to 80 oz/day (1,920 to 2,400 ml/day)	64 to 80 oz/day (1,920 to 2,400 ml/day)			Needs increase with higher temperature and humidity; higher level of activity; and consumption of alcohol, caffeine, and soda.

Nutrient	General recommendations	Recommendations for athletes	Food sources	Why do we need these?	Considerations
VITAMINS AND MINERALS					
Calcium	1,200 mg/day	1,200 to 1,500 mg	Low-fat milk and dairy products, parmesan and ricotta cheese, beans, tofu, canned salmon, dark leafy greens	Helps guard against osteoporosis, may result in weight loss or prevention of weight gain	Experts believe that calcium should be obtained from food sources. Some women (vegans, for example) may require supplementation.
Iron	8 mg/day	8 mg/day	Red meat, dark leafy greens, clams	Aids hemoglobin function (needed for oxygen consumption), proper immune function, and energy metabolism	Athletes training more than 6 hours per week should have their iron checked annually. Excessive amounts of iron are associated with heart disease and colon cancer.
Magnesium	320 mg/day	320 to 350 mg/day	Wheat germ, nuts, rye, soybeans, figs, almonds (1 oz, or 28 g = 77 mg), cashews, escarole, kale, and wheat bran	May ease irritability, anxiety, mood swings, insomnia; helps bones absorb calcium; raises high-density lipoprotein cholesterol (HDL-C) (good cholesterol); and lowers low-density lipoprotein cholesterol (LDL-C) (bad cholesterol)	Endurance and ultraendurance athletes should consume higher amounts.
Potassium	New recommendations being established	200 to 500 mg/day	Fruits, vegetables, whole grains	Aids in muscle hydration and recovery from fatigue	Potassium overload can have a toxic effect on the heart.
Selenium	55 µg/day	55 to 70 µg/day	Brazil nuts, beans, bran, garlic, mushrooms, and seafood	Benefits the immune system and helps repair daily cellular damage	
Sodium	New recommendations being established	1,000 to 4,000 mg/day	Salted foods (e.g., pretzels), celery, canned soups	Helps prevent dehydration	Ultraendurance athletes should consume 100 to 300 mg per hour. These recommendations need to be modified if a person has a medical condition that requires salt restriction.
Zinc	8 mg/day	8 to 12 mg/day	Bran, fish, wheat germ, yeast	Aids in postexertion tissue repair and helps convert food to fuel	

(continued)

Table 3.5 *(continued)*

Nutrient	General recommendations	Recommendations for athletes	Food sources	Why do we need these?	Considerations
Vitamin D	5 μg/day for women 9 to 50 years old, 10 μg/day for women 51 to 70 years old, 15 μg/day for women >70 years old	5 μg/day for women 9 to 50 years old, 10 μg/day for women 51 to 70 years old, 15 μg/day for women >70 years old	Sun (15 minutes per day), dairy products fortified with vitamin D, some fatty fish, orange juice fortified with vitamin D	Helps with calcium absorption and bone metabolism	Older people may not receive sufficient exposure to the sun, which can lead to osteopenia (generalized reduction in bone mass). In addition, those who live close to the polar regions do not get conversion of vitamin D on the skin from about November through March in the north and about May through September in the south. Thus, vitamin D intake is important. Some experts believe that the DRI for vitamin D needs to be increased.
Vitamin E	15 mg/day	15 to 100 mg/day	Olive oil, sunflower seeds, almonds, hazelnuts, salmon, wheat germ, asparagus, avocados, brown rice, egg yolks, lima beans, peas, sweet potatoes, vegetable oils (corn and soybean)	Antioxidant (prevents free radicals from building up, which can decrease risk of heart disease and cancer); protects the heart; may relieve hot flashes, breast tenderness, and vaginal dryness	Obtaining the recommended amount with food alone is difficult, so supplementation may be indicated. If a woman has a bleeding disorder or diabetes, or takes blood-thinning medication, she should check with her physician before supplementing.
Vitamin C	75 mg/day	75 to 500 mg/day	Strawberries, bell peppers, cantaloupe (rockmelon), kiwi, citrus fruits, and potatoes	Antioxidant, helps with immune function, as well as increased collagen	Athletes are encouraged to increase vitamin C intake from increased citrus fruit (e.g., oranges) consumption to prevent upper respiratory tract infection (URTI).
Vitamin A	700 μg/day	700 to 1,000 μg/day	Dark red and deep orange fruits and vegetables	Antioxidant, helps with eyesight	Athletes are encouraged to obtain beta-carotene from food sources first and to use natural marine sources (seaweed) if supplementation is needed.

NONNUTRIENTS

Nutrient	General recommendations	Recommendations for athletes	Food sources	Why do we need these?	Considerations
Lignans	No recommendations established	No recommendations established	Fruits, vegetables, whole grains, seeds containing lignans; flaxseeds are the best source of lignans.	A type of phytoestrogen. The body converts it to estrogen-like substances. Preliminary evidence suggests that lignans may ease hot flashes and vaginal dryness.	Flaxseeds should be ground and then sprinkled on cereals and yogurts, and added to baked goods and dressings. Consumption should be gradually increased, working up to 1 to 2 tsp per day. Adequate fluids must be consumed. Flaxseeds may cause gastrointestinal problems.

Nutrient	General recommendations	Recommendations for athletes	Food sources	Why do we need these?	Considerations
Omega-3 fatty acids	No recommendations established	No recommendations established	Fatty fish (twice per week). Mackerel, sardines, sockeye salmon, and rainbow trout have about 1,000 mg of omega-3 fatty acids in a 3.5 oz (about 90 g) serving. Flaxseeds and walnuts also contain omega-3 fatty acids.	Components of these fatty acids may protect against heart disease. They are believed to improve HDL-C while lowering triglyceride levels and blood pressure.	No DRI has been established for omega-3 fatty acids.
Phyto-estrogens	No recommendations established (research has suggested that about 30 mg/day is optimal).	No recommendations established (research has suggested that about 30 mg/day is optimal).	Soybeans, soy products, broccoli, carrots, citrus fruits, peppers, tomatoes, plums	Naturally occurring chemicals that behave like weak forms of human estrogen, phytoestrogens have the potential to diminish symptoms like hot flashes and vaginal dryness, and may guard against heart disease and osteoporosis.	If a woman has or has had estrogen-dependent cancer (like breast cancer), she should be careful about consuming excessive quantities of foods that contain natural estrogens.

[1]Amount of protein per pound (or per kilogram) depends on type, duration, frequency, and intensity of exercise. For example, a person new to weightlifting needs more protein than a veteran weightlifter does because the beginner will experience more muscle breakdown. A woman who exercises most days of the week at high intensity, lifts weights, and participates in aerobic activity needs more protein than one who performs low-level aerobic activity most days of the week.

[2]Monounsaturated fat is best because it decreases serum total cholesterol and low-density lipoprotein cholesterol (LDL-C) concentration yet may increase serum high-density lipoprotein (HDL-C) concentration. Monounsaturated fat should make up about 13% of total energy intake. Examples include olive oil, avocados, peanut butter, flaxseed, and some nuts. Polyunsaturated fat should make up about 10% of total energy intake, because it decreases serum total cholesterol and LDL-C concentration but may also decrease HDL-C concentration. Examples include soybean oil, sesame oil, and some nuts. Saturated fat should make up about 7% of total energy intake, because it increases serum total cholesterol and LDL-C concentration while also decreasing HDL-C concentration. Examples include animal fats such as lard, butter, and the fat within meats. Consumption of trans fat should be limited as much as possible. Trans fat results from the hydrogenation of foods to achieve longer shelf life and a mouth feel similar to that of butter. Trans fat increases serum total cholesterol and LDL-C concentration while lowering HDL-C concentration.

From S.L. Volpe, S.B. Sabelawski, and C.R. Mohr, 2007, *Fitness nutrition for special dietary needs* (Champaign, IL: Human Kinetics).

PHYSICAL ACTIVITY

Although diet is extremely important for maintaining quality of life for women as they approach and enter menopause, it is more effective when combined with exercise. Exercising 3 to 4 days per week will help reduce risk of CVD. Exercise can be aerobic (for example, walking) or anaerobic (for example, low-intensity weightlifting).

Benefits of Exercise for Menopausal Women

Exercise can decrease stress, which helps decrease LDL-C levels as well. Because weight gain often occurs during menopause because of both slower metabolism and lower energy expenditure, exercise is useful in helping to maintain a healthy body weight and normal blood pressure (less than 140/90 mmHg), further minimizing the risk of CVD. Moreover, an increase in abdominal fat (for example, taking on an apple shape) has been shown to increase the risk for type 2 diabetes mellitus, hypertension, and high blood lipid levels. Thus, a combination of more healthful eating and increased physical activity will greatly reduce the risk for CVD. Clearly, then, you should urge your older female clients to add both aerobic and resistance training to their regular regimens. The information that follows will be useful in showing them how to do so safely.

Benefits Common to Aerobic and Resistance Exercise

Menopausal women should exercise for a number of reasons. Exercise improves cardiovascular and aerobic endurance, strength, and flexibility, and it maintains or improves balance. Maintaining balance as one ages is extremely important. Those who have reasonable balance are less likely to fall when performing activities of daily living, such as reaching for a bowl in a high cupboard. Prevention of falls can save many lives each year. Older people, especially women, who fall may suffer a broken hip or spine, and they may never recover or may die from complications of surgery. There is a 12% to 20% risk of death following a hip fracture (Melton et al., 1998).

Aerobic and resistance exercise during menopause offers several additional benefits:

- Reduces adiposity (minimizing weight gain)
- Improves blood lipid levels and glucose levels (lowering risk of cardiovascular disease and diabetes mellitus, respectively)
- Improves blood pressure, enhances quality of sleep, and helps maintain bone mineral density
- Postpones the decline in central nervous system processing, thus maintaining or improving reaction time
- Improves or postpones the decline in fine and gross motor skills
- Decreases stress, anxiety, or depression; enhances mood; and improves self-esteem
- Empowers the exerciser, enhances social interactions (especially if people exercise in pairs or groups), and leads to new friendships (Bass, 2001)

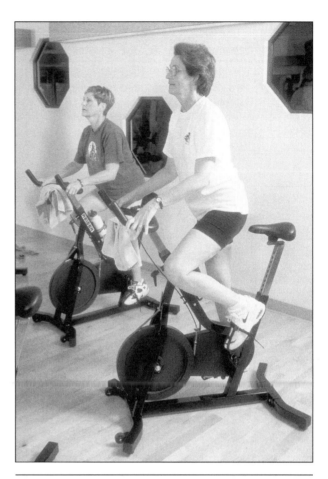

These women are addressing the cardiopulmonary aspect of strength. They will do well to include a resistance training component to their exercise regimen if they have not already done so.

Benefits Exclusive to Resistance Training

Weight-bearing exercise is uniquely important for minimizing bone loss during menopause. Dr. Miriam Nelson at Tufts University studied the effects of low-level weight training (using bands and ankle weights) on the bone mineral density of women 75 years of age and older. This low-level weight training, which can be performed at home, was able to prevent bone loss in these women when performed only 2 days per week. Preventing bone loss is especially important in the menopausal years, when bone mineral density can decrease dramatically. Strength training can also maintain or increase muscle mass, which may increase a person's metabolism at rest. Metabolism will rise because muscle is an active tissue that requires more energy to maintain,

Myths About Exercise During Menopause

People used to think that exercise during menopause was not healthy, that exercise would result in more hot flashes because energy expenditure increases body temperature. Fortunately, this myth has been debunked. Clearly, both aerobic and resistance exercise are important for a woman's health—before, during, and after menopause. Exercise not only helps prevent the weight gain often associated with menopause but also helps prevent an increase in blood lipid levels and helps maintain bone mineral density, typically preventing osteoporosis (in conjunction with a healthy diet and lifestyle that includes taking in sufficient calcium and not smoking). Dr. Miriam Nelson at Tufts University has written a number of wonderful books that address how women can increase their bone density by performing low-level weight training in their homes. Although healthy nutrition and exercise may not always prevent the increase in lipid levels associated with decreased *estrogen* levels during menopause, they can help keep the medication dose lower and maintain better overall health.

even at rest. Strength training can also decrease body fat, improve glucose tolerance (helping to prevent type 2 diabetes mellitus), decrease blood lipid levels and blood pressure (helping to prevent heart disease), and decrease gastro-intestinal transit time, which means that foods do not sit in the intestines for a long period, thus helping to prevent colon cancer and diverticulitis. Properly prescribed strength training will usually improve lower-back health and decrease pain from arthritis.

You may want to direct clients to refer to Dr. Nelson's book *Strong Women Stay Young* for more explanation about how to incorporate resistance training into their weekly schedule.

Exercise Prescription Guidelines

Before beginning any exercise program, clients should have a complete physical from a physician and obtain sound advice from an exercise physiologist (preferably, a clinically registered exercise physiologist), an exercise specialist, or a certified personal trainer. The trainer should be certified through the American College of Sports Medicine, the National Strength and Conditioning Association, or other reputable organization. Be aware that many online certifications are not reputable, so make sure that your clients know which certifying organizations are reliable.

A well-trained certified exercise physiologist will conduct an assessment to determine a specific exercise prescription for each person. The assessment involves determining a person's health status (with the help of her primary care physician), her current level of fitness (conducted through a stress test on a treadmill and various weight-training tests), and her previous exercise experience. The exercise physiologist or certified personal trainer and client will then establish the client's goals.

Although exercise prescriptions need to be individualized, the general recommendation is to accumulate at least 30 minutes per day of exercise on most days of the week to achieve cardiovascular benefits. If weight loss is a goal, most people will need to exercise more than 200 minutes per week, which would equate to 30 minutes per day every day or more than 30 minutes per day for 5 to 6 days per week (Jakicic, Winters, Lang, & Wing, 1999). A woman can perform this 30 or more minutes in a single bout or in shorter bouts throughout the day, if that works better for her schedule. Multiple bouts of exercise improve cardiovascular function and result in weight loss equally as well as one longer bout of exercise does (Jakicic et al.). The type of exercise that a woman performs depends on what she enjoys doing. If she enjoys walking, then that should be the preferred mode of exercise. But engaging in a variety of activities is important for several reasons: (1) variety helps maintain interest in exercise, (2) variety will typically lead to use of a greater number of muscles, and (3) variety helps prevent overuse injuries, which are often associated with repetitive motions. Furthermore, exercise in the morning produces the same benefits as exercise in the evening. The usual recommendation is to exercise early in the day simply because schedules tend to fill up during the day, making exercise later in the day less likely to happen. Table 3.6 offers a sample exercise prescription. Remember that these general guidelines will require modification for each person.

Table 3.6 Sample Exercise Prescription for Menopausal Women

Activity	When?	How long and at what intensity?	Why?
Stretching	Lightly before a workout. The best method is to walk slowly for a while before stretching. Stretching after exercise is more important than stretching before exercise. The muscles have been warmed up, so they stretch more readily.	About 10 minutes before exercise and about 15 to 20 minutes after exercise, at low intensity.	Helps with warm-up and cool-down. Maintains or increases flexibility. Helps maintain or improve balance.
Aerobic activity	Whatever time of day works best. Meal consumption should occur no later than 1 hour before activity to prevent excessive blood flow to the stomach. At least 3 days per week, but 5 days provides more consistency. Taking at least 1 day a week off from heavy training is necessary and will improve performance.	For a minimum of 30 minutes, typically at 60% to 80% of a person's predicted maximum heart rate, which is estimated by subtracting age from 220. Multiplying that number by 60% and 80% gives a heart rate range. The person should stay within that range during exercise activities.	Can improve overall health, prevent chronic disease, and maintain body weight.
Strength training	Whatever time of day works best. Meal consumption should occur no later than 1 hour before activity to prevent excessive blood flow to the stomach. Two days per week provides benefits. Competitive athletes who have goals different from simply maintaining health may need to train 3 to 4 days per week.	Depends on the number of muscles being worked on, but 30 minutes is typically enough for those who want to improve strength and bone mineral density. Eight to 12 repetitions on one piece of equipment, or more repetitions if using lighter weights or bands. One set of 8 to 12 repetitions is enough, but two sets are fine as well.	Can improve overall health, prevent chronic disease, and maintain body weight.

From S.L. Volpe, S.B. Sabelawski, and C.R. Mohr, 2007, *Fitness nutrition for special dietary needs* (Champaign, IL: Human Kinetics).

CASE STUDY

The case study from our guest dietitian (one of our authors, Chris Mohr) for this chapter focuses on a woman who was able to use lifestyle changes to delay medication for high blood lipid levels and then keep the dose low after she was required to take the medication.

L.M. was a 50-year-old woman who was physically active most of her life. She was diagnosed with *dyslipidemia* at a younger age, but her blood lipid levels were now under control through diet and exercise alone (that is, she took no medications). She had a body weight within normal range for her height; she was 64 in. (163 cm) tall and weighed 130 lb (59 kg). During perimenopause, she began to notice the following symptoms: hot flashes, mood swings, and weight gain. After routine blood work, she also learned that her blood triglyceride levels were now elevated to 450 mg per dl (normal levels are less than 150 mg per dl).

Her gynecologist suggested hormone replacement therapy to control her side effects and Tricor to decrease her serum triglyceride levels to within normal limits. She was reluctant to begin hormone replacement therapy because of the negative media reports that she had heard; thus, she opted to visit a registered dietitian as a first step. She also chose to try other dietary and exercise measures before taking a prescription medication, hoping that she could control her lipid levels with additional lifestyle changes instead of medication.

After reviewing her food records, we discussed some foods that she should consider limiting in her diet and others that she should increase. For example, L.M. routinely ate a breakfast of white toast with margarine and jelly and 1 cup (240 ml) of orange juice. We discussed the importance of including a variety of whole grains rather than refined grains and mentioned the possibility of choosing whole fruit rather than juice. I suggested that she switch from her white bread to higher-fiber bread; she chose one that had 3 g of fiber per slice. She likes cottage cheese, so rather than spreading jam on her toast each morning, she spread 1/2 cup (70 g) of low-fat cottage cheese on her toast. She was not aware that 8 oz (240 ml) of juice was equivalent to two servings of fruit, so she decided to switch to having one whole piece of fruit, such as an orange, apple, or other fruit that she likes.

She also started eating a salad each day for lunch, topped with canned salmon or fresh salmon, for the healthy omega-3 fatty acids and protein, along with other vegetables of choice and some type of legume, such as black beans or chickpeas. With her salads and sometimes at other times during the day, L.M was also sure to include low-fat soy milk.

She continued her traditional exercise routine, which included a minimum of 50 minutes of aerobic activity most days of the week and approximately 30 minutes of resistance training 3 days per week. She made an effort to increase her activity during routine daily events as well, so rather than calling an office mate or meeting with a friend for coffee, she would walk down the hall or suggest to her friend that they talk while taking a walk. These activities were in addition to her regular physical activity routine, because otherwise she had an inactive day. To track her progress, I suggested that she buy a pedometer. She could then monitor the number of steps that she took each day. If she did not achieve the recommended 10,000 steps, she could set aside some time at the end of the day to reach that level.

Inevitably, she gained a few pounds (a kilogram or so), but she was able to control this weight gain with her increased physical activity and the positive dietary changes. Little changes such as switching from 8 oz (240 ml) of fruit juice (two servings of fruit) to one whole piece of fruit per day not only reduced her energy intake but also helped keep her satiated for a longer period.

Her serum triglyceride levels ultimately decreased a small amount but could not be controlled solely through the diet and exercise regimen. She accepted the explanation that hormones are sometimes so powerful than they cannot be controlled naturally. She is now taking a very low dose of Tricor and maintaining the positive lifestyle changes that we discussed to keep that dose low and maintain her overall health.

Christopher R. Mohr, PhD, RD
President, Mohr Results, Inc.
Louisville, Kentucky

Pregnancy

Pregnancy is often one of the most wonderful times in a woman's life, but it does not come without challenges and complications. One of the challenges for a pregnant woman is to maintain a healthy diet and continue to be physically active, especially if she is experiencing some of the unpleasant side effects of pregnancy, such as nausea, vomiting, or heartburn.

PHYSIOLOGICAL CHANGES DURING PREGNANCY

Pregnancy results in many physiological changes because of the metabolic demands of the growing fetus. The cardiovascular system adapts to this situation in many ways. First, plasma volume increases by 40% to 50%. Cardiac output, the volume of blood that the heart pumps per minute, increases from about 5 L per minute prepregnancy to about 9 L per minute at 36 to 39 weeks (Ciliberto & Marx, 1998). In addition, blood pressure may decrease during the first two trimesters, but it usually returns to baseline in the third trimester. Pregnant women may also experience edema (a normal condition during pregnancy in which fluid accumulates in tissues or extremities). Because of the hormonal changes

of the mother and to accommodate the growing fetus, changes also occur in the respiratory tract (greater oxygen requirements may cause a pregnant woman to experience shortness of breath), gastrointestinal tract (nausea and vomiting typically occur during the first trimester, appetite increases during the second trimester, and pregnant women may experience food aversions, cravings, constipation, and heartburn), and kidneys (Mahan & Escott-Stump, 2004).

When a woman becomes pregnant, mechanical changes related to weight gain (increases in breasts, uterus, and fetus) result in a reallocation in a woman's center of gravity, which may result in problems with balance. This circumstance can lead to problems with certain types of exercise. Maternal temperature increases during exercise and pregnancy, and fetal temperature rises during maternal exercise. Some animal studies have shown that this increase in temperature due to exercise increases congenital abnormalities, but no evidence to date indicates that exercise in humans will result in congenital abnormalities in their babies (Wang & Apgar, 1998). Although it appears that, in humans, exercise is beneficial to pregnancy, the number of well-controlled studies in this area is lacking. Nonetheless, Kramer and McDonald (2006) recently published a review on the research that has been conducted in pregnant women who exercise. They searched the Cochrane Pregnancy and Childbirth Group's Trials Register (June 2005), MEDLINE (1966 to 2005 January week 1), EMBASE (1980 to 2005 January week 1), Conference Papers Index (earliest to 2005 January week 1), contacted researchers in the field, and searched reference lists of retrieved articles. They concluded that regular aerobic exercise during pregnancy appears to improve physical fitness. Nonetheless, available data are not sufficient to surmise important risks or benefits for the mother or fetus. Additional well-controlled trials are required before definitive recommendations can be made (Kramer & McDonald).

NUTRITION

The Dietary Reference Intakes (DRIs) for energy needs during pregnancy increase 150 kcal (627 kJ) per day during the first trimester and then rise to 350 kcal per day (1,463 kJ) during the second and third trimesters. If a woman also exercises, her energy needs will increase above those required for pregnancy (Wang & Apgar, 1998). The increase in energy needed for exercise will depend on the type, intensity, frequency, and duration of the activity. Supplementation, especially for iron and folic acid, are typically provided by the physician during pregnancy. A woman's folic acid needs double during pregnancy, and her iron needs often increase as well, especially in the later stages of pregnancy (Araujo, 1997; Orr, 1999). Figure 4.1 provides a food pyramid that will be useful for your pregnant clients. Here are more details about nutritional issues during pregnancy:

- **Folate**. Folate needs increase for pregnant women to prevent neural tube defects (in which the child is born with an underdeveloped brain or no brain at all, known as anencephaly) or

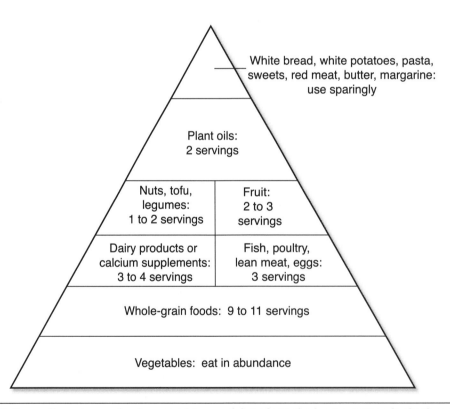

Figure 4.1   The Motherwell pregnancy food pyramid is a useful guide to the best nutrition for both mother and baby.

From S.L. Volpe, S.B. Sabelawski, and C.R. Mohr, 2007, *Fitness nutrition for special dietary needs* (Champaign, IL: Human Kinetics). Reprinted, by permission, from B. Berk, 2004, *Motherwell maternity fitness plan* (Champaign, IL: Human Kinetics), 56.

spina bifida (in which the spinal cord does not completely close) and to promote normal growth of the fetus and placenta. The Dietary Reference Intake (DRI), established as a Recommended Dietary Allowance (RDA), for folate is 600 mg per day. At least 400 mg of that should be derived from fortified foods or supplementation because folate from those sources is better absorbed in the body. Some rich food sources of folate are fortified cereals, lentils, spinach, asparagus, and broccoli (Mahan & Escott-Stump, 2004).

• **Iron**. As the maternal blood supply increases, the need for iron also increases. The RDA for iron for pregnant women is 27 mg per day (Tolerable Upper Intake Level, or UL = 45 mg per day). Iron supplementation is usually recommended and often needed to prevent iron deficiency. Many obstetric and gynecology practitioners prescribe a multivitamin supplement with iron. Iron absorption is enhanced when consumed with vitamin C. For example, a glass of orange juice taken with a multivitamin with iron will increase absorption of the iron. Coffee and tea should not be consumed with iron because the tannins in these beverages interferes with iron absorption (Mahan & Escott-Stump, 2004).

• **Nausea and vomiting**. As mentioned previously, one of the complications of pregnancy is nausea and vomiting. Pregnant women can consume certain foods to minimize nausea and vomiting, but the bottom line is that women should eat and drink what they can tolerate. If a woman continues to experience nausea and vomiting and is unable to consume adequate energy, she should contact her obstetrician or gynecologist. Some ways to avoid or minimize nausea and vomiting during pregnancy are to minimize smells (perhaps by having meals cooked or prepared outside the house), to consume saltines or carbonated beverages when nauseated, and to consume (sip) ginger ale. Some women have found it helpful to have a package of saltines by the bed and to eat a few crackers before getting up because nausea is often the worst in the morning. Pregnant women should continue to take their multivitamin with iron, especially if food intake is decreased.

• **Contraindicated practices**. The following should be avoided during pregnancy:

- Taking herbal preparations, which are not regulated by the federal government, can be dangerous because the purity of these products cannot be guaranteed. In addition, some herbs can cause miscarriages. Thus, a pregnant woman should avoid these preparations.

- Vitamin megadosing is also dangerous. Even one megadose of vitamin A could lead to birth defects. The pregnant woman should rely on her physician's recommendations regarding vitamin supplementation.

- Dieting should be avoided. Pregnancy is not the time for a woman to lose weight. Weight gain guidelines differ based on prepregnancy body weight.

- Consuming too much caffeine is unwise because caffeine can cross the placenta. Pregnant women should seek advice from their obstetrician or gynecologist about how much caffeine they can consume.

- Pregnant women should not drink alcohol at all. Consuming it can lead to fetal alcohol syndrome (FAS). Even small doses of alcohol can prevent oxygen delivery through the umbilical cord, causing brain damage, retarded growth, facial and vision abnormalities, and low Apgar scores.

- Smoking restricts blood supply to the fetus, limiting oxygen and nutrient delivery and removal of waste, slows growth, retards physical development, and could lead to low weight at birth. Even secondhand smoke can contribute to problems.

• **Hypoglycemia**. Because a pregnant woman experiences nausea and vomiting, especially during the first trimester, she must not allow her blood glucose levels to decrease. Eating small, frequent meals will help prevent nausea and vomiting and will help maintain blood glucose concentrations so that the future mother does not feel lightheaded or faint. In spite of such precautions, some women contract gestational diabetes during pregnancy. See the chapter on diabetes (chapter 7) for more information on this topic.

Weight Gain in Pregnancy

- Maternal uterus and breasts: 1.8 to 2.7 kg (4 to 6 lb)
- Maternal fat stores: 2.7 to 3.6 kg (6 to 8 lb)
- Blood supply: 1.8 to 2.7 kg (4 to 6 lb)
- Fetus and infant: 3.2 to 3.6 kg (7 to 8 lb)
- Amniotic fluid and placenta: 1.8 to 2.7 kg (4 to 6 lb)

- **Eating for healthy weight gain.** Weight gain during pregnancy is generally within the range of 11 to 18 kg (25 to 40 lb). The amount of weight that should be gained for a safe, healthy pregnancy is based on the prepregnancy body mass index (BMI), and recommendations made accordingly are listed in table 4.1 (Mahan & Escott-Stump, 2004). The section *"Weight Gain in Pregnancy"* lists how the weight gain in a typical, healthy pregnancy is distributed. A healthful meal plan would include eating approximately six times throughout the day, incorporating a variety of foods in each small meal. Pregnant women should avoid too many high-fat or high-sugar foods and should focus on obtaining adequate amounts of fruits, vegetables, whole grains, lean protein, and low-fat dairy sources. Low-fat and skim milk, cheese and yogurts, and lean meats such as chicken, turkey, and other lean meats or

protein substitutes are recommended. Artificial sweeteners should be avoided during pregnancy. A pregnant woman will gain more health benefits from water, milk, and juice than she will from artificially sweetened drinks.

NUTRITION-RELATED ISSUES IN PREGNANCY AND LACTATION

Adequate nutrition during and after pregnancy is not simply a matter of knowing what to eat and what not to eat. To meet the needs of her situation, a pregnant or lactating woman will have to translate that knowledge into practice and find time for the exercise that will enable her to metabolize her food for the most benefit. Read on for some practical tips.

Pregnant women who already have young children may find it difficult to consume any food at all during the day, let alone healthy meals! Nonetheless, a pregnant woman who already has other children, or is employed full time, or both, must be able to eat well and engage in adequate exercise. Doing so will ensure proper growth and development of the fetus as well as promote energy and good quality of life for the mother. Here are some tips to pass on to your clients:

- Have snacks when your young children are eating their snacks. Their snacks and your snacks can be the same healthy foods, and

Table 4.1 Weight-Gain Recommendations Based on Prepregnancy Body Mass Index (BMI)[1]

BMI category (kg/m^2)	First trimester kg (lb)	Second and third trimesters kg/week (lb/week)	Total kg (lb)
Underweight (BMI < 19.8)	2.3 (5)	0.49 (1.07)	12.5 to 18 (28 to 40)
Normal weight (BMI = 19.8 to 26)	1.6 (3.5)	1.6 (0.97)	11.5 to 16 (25 to 35)
Overweight (BMI = 26 to 29)	0.9 (2)	0.9 (2)	7 to 11.5 (15 to 25)
Obese (BMI > 29)			<7 (<15)

[1]For obese women who are pregnant, there are no recommendations for first-, second-, and third-trimester weight gain, but overall weight gain should not exceed the total weight gain listed. As with most guidelines, a woman should discuss her individual weight-gain requirements with her physician.

From S.L. Volpe, S.B. Sabelawski, and C.R. Mohr, 2007, *Fitness nutrition for special dietary needs* (Champaign, IL: Human Kinetics). Adapted from L.K. Mahan and S. Escott-Stump, 2004, *Krause's food, nutrition, & diet therapy* (Philadelphia, PA: WB Saunders Co.).

Sample Meal Plan for Pregnant Women

The sample meal plans provided in each chapter offer general guidelines that relate to the focus of the chapter. Providing sample meal plans for the vast number of scenarios suggested in each chapter would create a book of unmanageable length. Thus, we have provided sample guidelines with the hope that these will spark ideas for other meal plans. See tables A.1 through A.4 in the appendix for alternative food choices.

Breakfast

- 1 cup of Raisin Bran or whole-grain cereal = 60 g
- 1 cup of skim milk = 240 ml
- 1 1/4 cup of strawberries = 75 g
- 1 cup of orange juice or other 100% juice = 240 ml

Snack

- 8 small whole-wheat cracker squares = 80 g
- 2 tbsp of peanut butter = 30 g
- 12 oz of water = 360 ml

Lunch

- Egg salad sandwich
  - 1/2 cup of egg salad = 110 g
  - 2 slices of whole-wheat bread = 80 g
  - 2 slices each of lettuce and tomato = 30 g
  - 2 tsp of mayonnaise = 10 g
- 1 cup of mixed greens salad = 30 g
- 1 tbsp of vinaigrette dressing = 15 g
- 8 oz of skim milk = 240 ml

Snack

- 1 medium pear, orange, or apple = 80 g
- 1/4 cup of cottage cheese or 1 oz of low-fat cheese = 28 g
- 12 oz of water = 360 ml

Dinner

- 3 oz of roasted turkey breast or chicken breast (without skin) = 85 g
- 1/2 cup of butternut squash or peas = 110 g
- 1 small baked potato, 1/3 cup of rice, or 1/2 cup of pasta = 120 g
- 2 tsp of butter or margarine = 10 g
- 8 oz of skim milk = 240 ml

Snack

- 4 oz of vanilla low-fat yogurt = 110 g
- 3/4 cup of mixed berries (blueberries, blackberries, raspberries) = 170 g
- 3 graham crackers (1 square each) = 10 g
- 12 oz of water = 360 ml

This sample meal plan provides at least 100% of the Dietary Reference Intakes (DRIs) for energy, protein, fiber, vitamins A, C, E, B_6, B_{12}, thiamin, riboflavin, niacin, folate, calcium, iron, magnesium, phosphorus, zinc, and approximately

- 2,600 kcal (10,868 kJ),
- 117 g of protein,
- 100 g of fat,
- 31 g of fiber, and
- 3,900 mg of sodium.

From S.L. Volpe, S.B. Sabelawski, and C.R. Mohr, 2007, *Fitness nutrition for special dietary needs* (Champaign, IL: Human Kinetics).

eating with your children will allow for some pleasant downtime together.

- When your children are busy playing or taking a nap, use that time to ensure that you are consuming all the energy and varied nutrients that you need by having another snack or small meal. You can also use this time to perform some light exercise within the home.
- Furthermore, play with your children when they are playing! This sort of physical activity will accumulate throughout the day, and

the shorter bouts may be perfect, especially later in pregnancy.

Breast feeding is a wonderful experience for a mother to have with her new infant, and mother's milk provides the infant with an excellent source of antibodies and nutrients. The woman who is lactating needs more energy than when she was pregnant, because her energy expenditure for milk production and milk letdown (that is, when a woman is actually breast-feeding her infant) is quite high. The DRIs for pregnant women of any age increase from 175 g of carbohydrate per day

Myths About Energy Needs for Pregnant Women

Pregnant women often state that they are eating for two. Many gain weight too rapidly because their energy intake is much greater than their energy needs. In reality, the fetus needs only about 300 kcal to maintain metabolic homeostasis. Maintaining physical activity during pregnancy is important for the health of both the pregnant woman and the fetus. Taking in more energy than needed can have negative effects on the woman (for example, gestational diabetes), which could also have an effect on the child (above-normal birth weight). Therefore, pregnant women should be sure to stay within the normal, healthy weight-gain ranges to ensure a healthy pregnancy and a healthy baby.

during pregnancy to 271 g per day during lactation. Protein needs remain the same during pregnancy and lactation (71 g per day). The difference in carbohydrate needs equates to 384 kcal (1,605 kJ) more per day during lactation compared with pregnancy. Women who exercise will need to consume more energy per day to maintain body weight. For the most part, nutrient needs are greater for lactating women, as well. For energy and nutrient needs refer to the DRI tables at www.iom.edu/object.file/master/21/372/0.pdf. The tips for ensuring good nutrition and exercise given in the preceding paragraph are as applicable to lactating women as they are to pregnant women.

PHYSICAL ACTIVITY

Being physically active throughout life reduces disease risk and improves quality of life. Exercising during pregnancy is also beneficial, but a woman should use caution when beginning an exercise program during pregnancy because of the stress on the fetus. The following sections help guide the pregnant woman to exercise in a manner that is safe and healthy for her and her growing fetus.

Benefits of Exercise

The benefits of exercising during pregnancy are similar to those that occur when a woman is not pregnant. These include improved cardio-

vascular function that helps with the increased plasma volume during pregnancy, less overall weight gain, easier and less complicated labor, more rapid recovery after labor, and improved overall fitness (ParentsPlace.com, 2000; Mihailov, 2002). Furthermore, moderate exercise during pregnancy can lower the risk of serious complications (for example, increased blood pressure) that can lead to *preeclampsia*. Exercise during pregnancy can also decrease the risk of back problems and other musculoskeletal problems that are typically associated with weight gain during pregnancy. This preventive effect is often a result of increased strength and better posture (ParentsPlace.com; Palkhivala, 2001).

Psychologically, exercise during pregnancy has been shown to improve attitude and mood, increase self-esteem, increase body awareness, and lower depression and anxiety (ParentsPlace.com, 2000, 2002; Mihailov, 2002). Finally, exercise during pregnancy has been reported to decrease chances of requiring a cesarean section, improve sleep quality, and increase energy levels (ParentsPlace.com, 2002). Moderate exercise may also help to stimulate fetal growth (Palkhivala, 2001).

Other benefits of exercise during pregnancy include feeling better (exercise releases endorphins, the naturally occurring chemicals that the brain produces during exercise); experiencing less constipation; reducing wear and tear on the joints, which become loosened during pregnancy because of hormonal changes; looking better, because exercise increases blood flow to the skin, which is why women really do glow during pregnancy; achieving better preparation for birth by having strengthened muscles and a stronger heart, which will ease the burden of labor through increased endurance and better control of breathing; and returning to prepregnancy weight more quickly (http://kidshealth.org/parent/nutrition_fit/fitness/exercising_pregnancy.html).

Safety Considerations

Many women are encouraged to continue exercising during pregnancy, and those who have not been exercising prepregnancy would likely benefit from incorporating some kind of low- to moderate-intensity exercise into their daily routine. Walking and swimming are safe, are not weight bearing, and will provide benefits to the pregnant woman and her fetus. Low- to moderate-intensity activities are best, but higher-intensity exercise may be safe for women who have been exercising at high intensity prepregnancy. None-theless, caution should be taken to ensure the safety of the fetus and the pregnant woman. A pregnant woman should consult with her obstetrician or gynecologist before starting an exercise regimen, even if she has been exercising. A woman who is a competitive athlete should consult with her obstetrician or gynecologist more frequently (for example, to monitor the fetus). The following are common questions (and respective answers) that people ask about the safety of exercise during pregnancy.

- **Is it safe for a woman who has become pregnant to begin exercise?** If a woman has not been exercising but chooses to do so after she has become pregnant, it typically is not harmful. First, however, she should discuss her exercise plan with her obstetrician or gynecologist and with an exercise physiologist or certified personal trainer who has expertise in exercise with pregnant women (Pivarnik, 1994). If a woman does begin to exercise during pregnancy, the exercise should be low impact, such as walking or swim-ming, and she should begin with shorter sessions until she is able to continue for longer periods (BabyCenter.com, 2002). Certainly, if a person was not a competitive athlete before pregnancy, pregnancy is not the time to begin a competitive program, but a woman can begin to exercise at low intensity. As stated earlier, walking and swimming are suitable low-impact activities for the pregnant woman, especially for the woman who was not active before pregnancy.

- **Should the trained athlete change her routine?** Even if a woman is well trained before her pregnancy, she may need to alter the intensity and type of activity if these could be harmful to her health and the health of the fetus. Because the change in weight distribution affects a pregnant woman's center of gravity, even a well-coordinated woman is likely to become less coordinated, increasing risk of falls. Thus, the American College of Obstetricians and Gynecologists (ACOG) recommends that pregnant women avoid sports that require excellent balance, such as bicycling, horseback riding, downhill skiing, or water skiing. Pilates and yoga are excellent ways

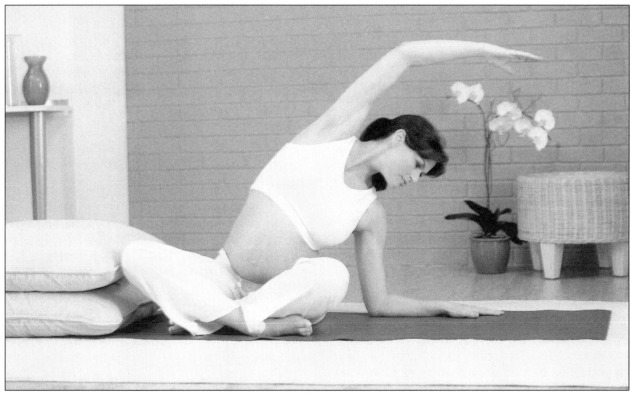

Yoga is an excellent form of exercise for pregnant women, provided that they are either already experienced in yoga techniques, or that they work with a certified yoga instructor.

© Jupiter Images

to help maintain balance, and they can be safely altered for the pregnant woman. Although the risk of engaging in activities that require good balance may seem small, the consequences can be devastating. For example, falling off a bicycle can result in premature labor, an abrupted placenta, or even death of the fetus. Nonetheless, the prepregnancy fitness of the pregnant woman, the trimester of pregnancy, and the intensity of the activity will determine the risk of falls and danger to the fetus (www.babycenter.com/expert/pregnancy/pregnancyfitness/7229.html). A good rule to observe is that if a woman is unsure whether she will be able to perform the activity safely, she should err on the side of caution.

• **Are there contraindications for exercise for some pregnant women?** If a woman is at risk for having preterm labor or intrauterine growth restriction, even if she was extremely active before her pregnancy, she should decrease her exercise intensity in the second and third trimesters (www.babycenter.com/expert/pregnancy/pregnancyfitness/7229.html). Although exercising during pregnancy offers many benefits, some contraindications exist. For example, women who have pregnancy-induced hypertension may not be able to exercise because the exercise will further increase blood pressure. But if closely monitored by a physician or trained exercise physiologist, a woman with pregnancy-induced hypertension may be able to tolerate shorter, lower-intensity bouts of exercise. Other contraindications to exercise include preterm rupture of membranes, preterm labor during the prior or current pregnancy or both, incompetent cervix or cerclage, persistent second- or third-trimester bleeding, and intrauterine growth retardation (Paradise Valley Community College, 2002). Because the contraindications are crucial to the health of both mother and child, they are summarized in the section *"Contraindications to Exercise During Pregnancy."*

• **Are certain exercise-related risks particularly heightened for pregnant women?** Dehydration, *hypovolemia* (low blood volume), and low blood pressure should all be avoided. Pregnant women should eat several times each day (meals and snacks) and drink adequate fluids, especially if they are active. Dehydration, hypovolemia, and hypotension can be prevented by not skipping meals and by hydrating adequately. Pregnant women need to be disciplined with their eating

---

Contraindications to Exercise During Pregnancy

Contraindications

- Pregnancy-induced hypertension
- Preterm rupture of membranes
- Preterm labor during the prior or current pregnancy
- Incompetent cervix or cerclage
- Persistent second- or third-trimester bleeding
- Placenta previa
- Intrauterine growth retardation

Relative contraindications

- Chronic hypertension
- Thyroid function abnormality
- Cardiac disease
- Vascular disease
- Pulmonary disease

Adapted from The American College of Obstetricians and Gynecologists, 2002, "ACOG Committee Opinion. Number 267: Exercise during pregnancy and the postpartum period," *Obstetrics and Gynecology* 99(1): 171-173.

---

and hydration habits, especially if they have younger children, a circumstance that may cause them to miss meals or consume foods on the run. For the most part, however, a woman who is already fit before pregnancy can typically continue her workouts during pregnancy without compromising her health or the health of her developing fetus (BabyCenter.com, 2002).

Guidelines for Exercise

The main goal is to exercise daily while avoiding activities that will result in excess pressure on the fetus or excess bouncing or pounding (see *"Activities to Avoid During Pregnancy"*). In general, women need to listen to their bodies more carefully while exercising during pregnancy. They should not exercise to the point of feeling their muscles burn. If a woman is feeling nauseous, dizzy, or weak, perhaps because of not consuming enough food and fluids during the day, she should cease the activity immediately, consume food and fluids, sit down or lie down, and elevate her feet. Of course, contacting her obstetrician or gynecologist may be necessary if this becomes frequent or more serious. Becoming more in tune with the body can be key to ensuring a proper balance of food and fluid intake and exercise. Women who have been competitive athletes before pregnancy are usually adept at listening to their bodies. Nonetheless, pregnant women with a history of medical problems, such as anemia, hypertension, diabetes mellitus, hyperthyroidism or hypothyroidism, or seizure disorders, to name a few, should exercise only with the approval of their health care provider and should be monitored even more closely during pregnancy (www. marchofdimes.com/professionals/681_1150. asp).

A woman who begins an exercise program during pregnancy should start slowly and only gradually increase intensity, duration, and frequency. Typically, later in pregnancy, shorter, multiple bouts of exercise are preferred for both the comfort of the pregnant woman and the safety of the fetus. Guidelines for warm-up and cool-down are the same for pregnant women as they are for other people. Refer to chapter 2, "Aging," for guidelines. Table 4.2 provides a list of exercises that are generally beneficial for pregnant women, along with the average energy expended.

Guidelines for Aerobic Exercise

A pregnant woman should generally not exercise above 60% of her maximal oxygen consumption ($\dot{V}O_2$max) (BabyCenter.com, 2002). To prevent overexertion, she should closely monitor her heart rate at preexercise, about every 10 minutes during exercise, as well as immediately postexercise and 10 to 15 minutes postexercise. The heart rate should not go above 140 beats per minute during exercise (BabyCenter.com), but

the target heart rate can be adjusted, depending on the person's fitness level and goals. Keep in mind that multiple short bouts of exercise can be

Activities to Avoid During Pregnancy

Activity or Exercise to Avoid
- Waterskiing
- Horseback riding
- Snowboarding
- Downhill skiing
- Surfing
- Tennis
- Bicycling
- Scuba and other pressurized sports[1]

Exercise-Related Activities to Avoid[2]
- Hot tubs and Jacuzzis
- Waterslides
- Amusement park rides

[1]Scuba and other pressurized sports should not be performed because air bubbles can form in the bloodstream as a person surfaces to the top.

[2]Although these are not exercises, many active individuals enjoy hot tubs or Jacuzzis after a workout. Pregnant women should avoid these throughout pregnancy because the heat can increase the risk of birth defects. Waterslides and amusement parks are dangerous because of the impact of landing in the water and the occasionally violent motion of rides.

From S.L. Volpe, S.B. Sabelawski, and C.R. Mohr, 2007, *Fitness nutrition for special dietary needs* (Champaign, IL: Human Kinetics). Adapted from www.babycenter.com/expert/pregnancy/pregnancyfitness/7229.html.

Table 4.2 Average Energy Expenditure of Activities Beneficial for Pregnant Women

Activity	Average kcal (kJ) expended
Walking 1 mi (1.6 km)	~150 (627)
Walking 2 mi (3.2 km)	~300 (1,254)
Swimming for 30 minutes	~200 (836)
Yoga for 60 minutes	~200 (836)
Pilates for 60 minutes	~235 (982)
Gardening for 60 minutes	~100 (418)

From S.L. Volpe, S.B. Sabelawski, and C.R. Mohr, 2007, *Fitness nutrition for special dietary needs* (Champaign, IL: Human Kinetics).

just as beneficial as a single long bout of exercise. If the pregnant woman is not able to sustain her exercise routine for a single longer bout, she should be encouraged to exercise in several shorter bouts, which will provide the same cardiovascular benefits. Monitoring the heart rate during pregnancy is important, because although the research in this area has provided mixed results, some studies have found that higher-intensity exercise may lead to premature birth or low birth weight. No definitive threshold for maximal heart rate during exercise in pregnancy has been established. Thus, although it may be cumbersome and even frustrating to take heart rates, especially for women who have been exercising before pregnancy, taking radial pulse every 10 minutes would be a good idea. For easier tracking, a pregnant woman can use a heart rate monitor to ensure that her heart rate does not exceed 140 beats per minute. Table 4.3 provides general guidelines for aerobic exercise while pregnant.

Guidelines for Resistance Training

Little research has been done on resistance training during pregnancy. Most of the exercise guidelines about beginning or continuing exercise during pregnancy are in reference to aerobic activity. Nonetheless, resistance training during pregnancy can be beneficial. If a woman has been performing resistance training before pregnancy, she can continue those activities but may need to reduce the intensity by performing more repetitions with less weight. Furthermore, as her center of gravity shifts, she may need to alter or discontinue some weight-training activities. During pregnancy, a woman should use weight-training machines rather than free weights because of the balance issue. Other strength-training activities that are appropriate during or after pregnancy are mat Pilates and using Therabands (note that Therabands are used in Pilates). These activities are excellent for increasing strength, place less pressure on the mother and fetus, and will not increase blood pressure as much as other kinds of strength-training activities will. Those who have been strength training before pregnancy may want to consider mat Pilates or using Therabands later in pregnancy. Benefits of weight training during pregnancy include decreasing common pregnancy discomforts, building strength for carrying the new baby, improving state of mind, and reducing stress (www.befitmom.com/strength_training.html). Regardless of the type of strength training that she performs during pregnancy, the pregnant woman must always

Table 4.3 Guidelines for Aerobic Exercise for Pregnant Women of Different Fitness Levels or With Different Conditions[1]

Fitness level or condition	Guidelines
Woman who has not been active at all before pregnancy	Low-intensity walking would be a perfect activity. Start slowly, even if only 5 minutes at a time or 5 minutes per day. Using Therabands for light resistance training would also be a good activity. Monitor heart rate.
Woman who has been moderately active before pregnancy	Maintain the moderate activity; adjust activity during each trimester as needed. If resistance training was not part of the exercise regimen before pregnancy, do not begin a program now, although using Therabands for resistance training would be an excellent activity. Monitor heart rate.
Woman who has been very active before pregnancy	Continue activities performed before pregnancy. If these included resistance training, decrease the amount of weight to decrease stress on the fetus but adjust the number of repetitions. Monitor heart rate.
Woman who is experiencing increased blood pressure or gestational diabetes	Perform activities of very low intensity, namely walking, for short periods throughout the day. If possible, perform longer bouts of walking to help with blood pressure and blood glucose control. Monitor heart rate, blood pressure, and blood glucose concentrations.

[1]All pregnant women should avoid dangerous activities listed earlier in the chapter.

maintain her balance to ensure her safety and the safety of the fetus.

CASE STUDY

The case study for this chapter involves a woman who was already physically active before pregnancy. Chris Mohr discusses how he was able to help his client regain her healthy lifestyle pattern during her pregnancy.

C.S. was a 28-year-old pregnant woman. She had no known health problems at the start of her pregnancy and was very active physically, having competed in many marathons and triathlons. Her main goal with her pregnancy was to gain the recommended 11 to 16 kg (25 to 35 lb) over 9 months, continue to be physically active as long as possible, and eat optimally for herself and her child.

During her first trimester, C.S. realized that she was having increasing difficulty running. She quickly became short of breath, her feet and knees ached, and her heart rate increased rapidly within a short time. She was discouraged and became anxious about attempting any other activities for fear that doing so would hurt the fetus. She continued to eat additional foods because she had a number of cravings. She began to lose her normal vigor, giving her a grim outlook on the entire pregnancy.

Within the first 2 months of her pregnancy, C.S. gained 11 kg (25 lb). Her physician sent her to me to discuss her eating and exercise habits. She was not having any health abnormalities other than the rapid weight gain. We met and talked about the types and quantity of foods that she was consuming and about her cravings. C.S. was a compliant patient because she was healthy, and her rapid weight gain was a big change for her. She knew that if she continued her present eating habits and sedentary behavior, she would ultimately hurt herself and potentially the fetus.

We revisited some exercise strategies that C.S. could potentially follow. Because she had recently competed in triathlons, she was comfortable in the water. Water activities are non-weight-bearing, so they would put less stress on her body. I suggested that she attempt a low-impact water aerobics class or swim laps in the pool. Because of her earlier experience with a rapid heart rate when initiating exercise, I suggested that she take her pulse regularly throughout her exercise sessions to ensure that the increase was slow and steady. I also recommended that she measure her heart rate after cessation of physical activity to ensure that it returned to resting levels. *ACSM's Resource Manual for Guidelines for Exercise Testing and Prescription* (American College of Sports Medicine, 2006) also suggests that during pregnancy, regular exercise on most days of the week is preferable to intermittent activity.

C.S. began monitoring her portion sizes more closely to ensure that she was not increasing her energy intake too much (not above the DRI recommendations). She also began going to the YMCA regularly and thoroughly enjoyed water aerobics and swimming laps. Her body weight began to stabilize, putting her back on track for the recommended weight gain. She also had more energy and a more positive outlook. Furthermore, she kept more healthful snack foods around the house, such as fruits, vegetables, yogurt, and whole-grain products.

Christopher R. Mohr, PhD, RD
President, Mohr Results, Inc.
Louisville, Kentucky

Vegetarianism

This chapter addresses people who exercise and are vegetarians. We will discuss the variations in the nutritional intake of several types of vegetarians. Many competitive athletes are vegetarians. Like those who are not vegetarians, people who eat a vegetable-based diet must maintain energy balance and take in the necessary nutrients.

BASICS OF VEGETARIANISM

Eating a more vegetable-based diet has been shown to decrease the risk of certain chronic diseases. Some of the many types of vegetarian diets, however, may not provide all the needed nutrients to be beneficial against chronic disease. Whether a person is a vegetarian or not, a healthy diet is required—one with variety, enough energy, and the proper amount of nutrients. These considerations are even more important for active people.

Types of Vegetarians

Before discussing the nutrition and exercise considerations for vegetarians, we need to define the different types of vegetarians. There are at least nine different types of vegetarians, some more strict in what they will eat than others. The

nine defined in this chapter are semivegetarian, pesco-vegetarian, vegetarian, lacto-ovo vegetarian, lacto-vegetarian, ovo-vegetarian, vegan (pronounced "vee-gan"), fruititarians, and macrobiotic vegetarians.

Semivegetarians eat fish, poultry, eggs, dairy products, fruits, vegetables, grains, legumes, and nuts, but they may exclude red meat from their diets or consume red meat only occasionally. Pesco-vegetarians consume all that a semivegetarian does, with the exception of poultry and red meat. Lacto-ovo vegetarians consume dairy products, eggs, vegetables, grains, legumes, fruits, and nuts, but they exclude meat, fish, and poultry from their diets. Lacto-vegetarians consume dairy products, vegetables, fruits, grains, legumes, and nuts but exclude meat, fish, poultry, and eggs from their diet. Ovo-vegetarians include eggs, vegetables, fruits, grains, legumes, and nuts but exclude meat, fish, poultry, and dairy products from their diets. Vegans consume only foods from plant sources: vegetables, fruits, legumes, grains, seeds, nuts. Vegans often do not consume honey because it is derived from bees. Many vegans do not buy anything that was manufactured using any sort of animal product (leather shoes, leather coats, and so forth). Of the vegetarians discussed thus far, vegans are the strictest in their practices.

Two other types of vegetarians that consume limited kinds of foods are fruitarians and those who consume a *macrobiotic diet*. Fruititarians consume only raw and dried fruits, nuts, and seeds in their diets. Those who consume macrobiotic diets basically begin as vegans but progressively eliminate more foods. Ultimately, they consume only brown rice and small amounts of water and herbal tea, although some people who practice macrobiotic diets may include fish and some vegetables. Strict fruitarian and macrobiotic diets are far too extreme to provide all the nutrients needed.

Although vegans can be extremely restrictive in their diets, they can be healthy if they include a variety of foods. But a vegetarian diet of any type that excessively restricts any food or groups of foods, without replacing those foods with a non-animal-derived substitute (for example, beans or hummus for meat), can lead to malnutrition and even death. The components of a well-balanced vegetarian diet include a variety of vegetables, fruits, whole grains, legumes, and nuts. That is, to enhance health, the vegetarian diet needs to be as varied and nutritious as a nonvegetarian diet. Numerous studies have shown that plant-based diets are healthier than meat-based diets in preventing and reducing cardiovascular disease,

diabetes, and cancer risk factors. Nonetheless, vegetarian diets that are deficient in nutrients and energy are not healthy, especially if they lead to protein malnutrition or protein-energy malnutrition (Sabate, 2003). For a summary of the different types of vegetarians, refer to table 5.1.

Benefits of Vegetarianism

The many benefits of becoming a vegetarian occur in those who consume a varied and well-balanced diet, a goal that is not difficult to achieve unless one is a fruititarian or practicing a macrobiotic diet, which are too limited to permit healthy consumption of a variety of foods. Other vegetarians, including vegans, have many choices, even in regular supermarkets, that allow them to consume most of the required nutrients. Vegans, who do not include any animal foods or foods from animals in their diets, often need to supplement with vitamin B_{12}, because this vitamin is derived solely from animal products. Some vegans, especially those who may not always be careful about consuming a variety of foods, may also benefit from calcium, iron, zinc, and vitamin D supplementation.

A number of epidemiological studies have assessed the benefits of a vegetarian diet and

Table 5.1   Types of Vegetarians at a Glance

	Eat meat	Eat poutry	Eat fish	Eat eggs	Eat dairy products	Eat legumes	Eat grains	Eat fruits	Eat vegetables	Eat nuts and seeds
Semivegetarians	X*	X	X	X	X	X	X	X	X	X
Pesco-vegetarians			X	X	X	X	X	X	X	X
Lacto-ovo vegetarians				X	X	X	X	X	X	X
Lacto-vegetarians					X	X	X	X	X	X
Ovo-vegetarians				X		X	X	X	X	X
Vegans						X	X	X	X	X
Fruititarians								X		X
Macrobiotic vegetarians							X**			

*Consume red meat occasionally.

**Begin as vegans and ultimately consume only brown rice, water, and herbal tea.

reported certain health benefits. Many of these studies have shown that vegetarians have lower incidence of heart disease, cancer, diabetes mellitus, hypertension, obesity, kidney stones, **gallstones,** and **diverticular disease**. Vegetarians gain these benefits because, in general, they consume moderate amounts of energy and protein, consume more fiber than the average person does, consume lower amounts of saturated fat and cholesterol, consume higher amounts of monounsaturated and polyunsaturated fats, and, because of their high fruit and vegetable consumption, have diets that are generally higher in antioxidants and phytochemicals compared with diets of the general population.

In addition, many vegetarians exercise regularly, do not smoke, and do not drink alcohol at all or drink in moderation. Alewaeters et al. (2005) reported that in a sample of 326 vegetarian men and women compared with more than 9,000 controls who were not vegetarians, body mass index (BMI; weight in kilograms divided by height in meters squared) was significantly lower in the vegetarians than it was in the control group. Vegetarians also smoked significantly less and were significantly more physically active than their nonvegetarian counterparts. Therefore, separating the effects of the vegetarian diet from the effects of the healthy overall lifestyle of vegetarians is difficult. Nonetheless, it is clear that a higher intake of plant protein (and more whole foods in general) will decrease risk of cardiovascular disease, diabetes, and some cancers, because of the lower intake of saturated fat, cholesterol, and animal protein and the higher consumption of complex carbohydrates, dietary fiber, and vitamins and minerals that also act as antioxidants (Leitzmann, 2005). Indeed, "Well-balanced vegetarian diets are appropriate for all stages of the life cycle, including children, adolescents, pregnant and lactating women, the elderly and competitive athletes" (Leitzmann). Furthermore, the position of the American Dietetic Association and Dietitians of Canada (2003) is that dietetics professionals must "support and encourage" and be respectful of people who consume vegetarian diets. The registered dietitian can play a primary role in educating people about the benefits of a healthy vegetarian diet and the risk of a poorly planned vegetarian diet.

In addition, the higher fiber content of a vegetarian diet helps control energy intake, which may be a benefit for some people. Athletes, however, typically have high needs for energy. Therefore, they may have difficulty consuming sufficient energy on a vegetarian diet. Plenty of athletes are vegetarians, however, so the dietitian must educate athletes about how to increase energy without too much added fiber (with fruit and yogurt smoothies and peanut butter, for example) to prevent bloating during competition.

Beneficial Properties of Plant Foods

Although we covered antioxidants and phytochemicals in the chapter about menopause, we offer here additional information about how plant foods can be beneficial in the prevention of chronic disease in vegetarians.

Antioxidants (also known as free radical scavengers) are substances in food that help fight infection and disease by protecting cells from the harmful effects of oxidation. Oxidation of lipids (polyunsaturated lipids, like those that surround cells in the body) occurs on a daily basis and produces free radicals. Free radicals are molecules in need of electrons, and they get them by stealing them from other molecules. This process may cause damage to the DNA of cells, which may result in cancer and heart disease. Nutrients such as vitamins C and E, beta-carotene, zinc, iron, and selenium can all act as antioxidants. Because most vegetarians consume higher amounts of plant foods, their natural consumption of the antioxidant nutrients is typically greater than that contained in the diet of the average person, resulting in greater protection from chronic disease.

Phytochemicals, literally "plant chemicals," are nonnutrient compounds in plant foods that protect against infection and disease. Phytochemicals also help prevent damage from free radicals, which can lead to certain cancers and heart disease and may be involved in the aging process. Over a thousand phytochemicals have been discovered, and estimates are that just one serving of vegetables may contain more than a hundred different phytochemicals (Polk, 1996).

Vegetarian diets have been shown to decrease the risk of cancer because of their high fruit and vegetable content (Block, Patterson, & Subar, 1992). More recently, Thompson and colleagues (2006) have reported that it may be more beneficial to consume a more diverse botanical diet that provides smaller amounts of more

Comparison of a Typical Nonvegetarian Diet Versus a Typical Vegetarian Diet

Nonvegetarian Diet

Breakfast

- 2 medium eggs = 60 g
- 2 slices of white toast = 160 g
- 2 tbsp of butter for toast = 30 g
- 1 cup of coffee = 240 ml
- 1 tbsp of cream = 15 g
- 2 tsp of sugar = 10 g

Lunch

- 1/4 lb of hamburger from a fast-food restaurant = 113 g of meat plus other ingredients
- 1 cup of french fries = 120 g
- 16 oz of regular soda = 480 ml

Snack

- 1 medium-size candy bar = 150 g
- 12 oz of regular soda = 360 ml

Dinner

- 2 oz of baked chicken breast = 60 g
- 1/2 cup of broccoli = 60 g
- 1 cup of white rice = 115 g
- 1 cup of canned peaches = 113 g
- 4 oz of red wine = 120 ml

Snack

- 2 cups of buttered popcorn = 220 g
- 8 oz of regular soda = 240 ml

The nonvegetarian diet provides, on average, 3,060 kcal (12,791 kJ); 5 g of fiber (about 1 g of soluble and 4 g of soluble fiber); and 40% of energy from total fat, including about 25% from saturated fat, 10% from polyunsaturated fat, and 5% from monounsaturated fat.

Vegetarian Diet (Vegan)

Breakfast

- 1 cup of whole grain cereal = 115 g
- 1/2 cup of calcium-fortified soy milk = 120 ml
- 1 cup of mixed berries (strawberries, blueberries, raspberries, blackberries) = 113 g
- 8 oz of orange juice = 240 ml

Lunch

- 1/2 cup of baked tofu = 60 g
- 1 cup of brown rice = 115 g
- 1 cup of steamed dark leafy green vegetables, such as kale, broccoli, bok choy = 115 g
- 1/2 of a medium banana = 40 g
- 1 medium red pear = 80 g
- 12 oz of water = 360 ml

Snack

- 8 whole-wheat cracker squares = 80 g
- 2 tbsp of natural peanut butter = 30 g
- 12 oz of water = 360 g

Dinner

- 1 cup of whole-wheat pasta = 120 g
- 1/2 cup of marinara sauce = 120 ml
- 1/4 cup of green peppers sauteed in 1 tbsp of olive oil = 60 g
- 1 tbsp of onions sauteed in 1 tbsp of olive oil = 20 g
- 1 cup of mixed greens salad = 110 g
- 2 tbsp of vinaigrette dressing (made with olive oil) = 30 g
- 8 oz of 100% juice = 240 ml

Snack

- 1 cup of low-fat plain soy yogurt = 113 g
- 1/2 cup of blueberries = 55 g
- 8 oz of water = 240 ml

The vegetarian diet provides, on average, 1,845 kcal (7,712 kJ); 25 g of fiber (about 12 g of soluble fiber and 13 g of insoluble fiber); and 25% of energy from total fat, including about 13% from monounsaturated fat, 9% from polyunsaturated fat, and 3% from saturated fat.

From S.L. Volpe, S.B. Sabelawski, and C.R. Mohr, 2007, *Fitness nutrition for special dietary needs* (Champaign, IL: Human Kinetics).

phytochemicals than to consume a less diverse botanical diet that contains greater amounts of fewer phytochemicals. Increasing awareness and promotion of vegetable foods as beneficial to health has resulted in the coining of terms to refer to such foods and their effects. See the section *"Catchphrases in Nutrition"* for some of these terms and their definitions. Emphasize to your clients that it is best to obtain a small amount of many phytochemicals each day rather than larger amounts of fewer phytochemicals.

Table 5.2 lists some of the most commonly studied phytochemicals. These are the compounds in the respective foods that assist in disease prevention. Remember, the best approach is to obtain a small amount of many phytochemicals each day as opposed to a larger amount of fewer phytochemicals.

Fiber is another component found in fruits, vegetables, and grains. Fiber comes in two forms: soluble and insoluble. Soluble fiber protects more against heart disease because it binds to fat and cholesterol in the intestines to decrease their absorption. An example of a soluble fiber is oat bran. Insoluble fiber aids in bowel regularity, resulting in less stools remaining in the intestines, which protects against colon cancer and diverticular disease. Insoluble fiber is found in wheat products. In most cases a person can get a good balance of soluble and insoluble fiber by consuming fruits, vegetables, and whole-grain products.

Table 5.2   Most Commonly Studied Phytochemicals

Food	Phytochemicals	Possible health benefits
Allium vegetables (garlic, onions, chives, leeks)	Allyl sulfides	May reduce risk of certain cancers (prostate, esophageal, stomach) and hypertension
Cruciferous vegetables (broccoli, cauliflower, cabbage, brussels sprouts, kale, turnips, bok choy, kohlrabi)	Indoles/glucosinolates, sulfaforaphane, isothiocyanates/ thiocyanates, thiols	May reduce risk of certain cancers (lung) and cardiovascular disease
Solanaceous vegetables (tomatoes, peppers)	Lycopene	May reduce risk of some cancers (ovarian, colon) and certain eye diseases
Umbelliferous vegetables (carrots, celery, cilantro, parsley, parsnips)	Carotenoids, phthalides, polyacetylenes	May reduce risk of certain cancers
Compositae plants (artichoke)	Silymarin	May reduce the risk of certain cancers (not recommended during pregnancy)
Citrus fruits (oranges, lemons, grapefruit), glucarates	Monoterpenes (limonene), carotenoids	May reduce risk of certain cancers and cardiovascular disease
Other fruits (grapes, berries, cherries, apples, cantaloupe [rockmelon], watermelon, pomegranate)	Ellagic acid, phenols, flavonoids (quercetin)	May reduce risk of heart disease
Beans, grains, seeds, (soybeans, oats, barley, brown rice, whole wheat, flaxseed), protease inhibitors	Flavonoids (isoflavones), phytic acid, saponins	May reduce risk of certain cancers and cardiovascular disease
Herbs, spices (ginger, mint, rosemary, thyme, oregano, sage, basil, turmeric, caraway, fennel)	Gingerols, flavonoids, monoterpenes (limonene)	May assist in improving digestive disorders
Licorice root, green tea, polyphenols	Glycyrrhizin catechins	May reduce risk of certain cancers and cardiovascular disease, and improve immune function

From S.L. Volpe, S.B. Sabelawski, and C.R. Mohr, 2007, *Fitness nutrition for special dietary needs* (Champaign, IL: Human Kinetics). Adapted from S. Dresbach and A. Rossi, Ohio State University Extension Fact Sheet [Online]. Available: http://ohioline.osu.edu/hyg-fact/5000/5050.html [August 1, 2006].

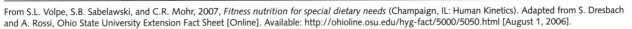

Catchphrases in Nutrition

chemoprevention—Use of one or more chemical compounds to prevent cancer.

designer foods—Foods that have been supplemented with substances high in disease-preventing compounds (Hasler et al., 2004).

functional food—Any altered food or food ingredient that may supply a health benefit above the traditional nutrients that it contains (Hasler et al.).

nutraceutical—Particular chemical compounds in food, including vitamins and additives, that may assist in prevention of chronic disease.

pharmafood—Food or nutrient that may assist with prevention and treatment of disease (Hasler et al.).

phytochemical—Nonnutritive plant chemicals composed of disease-preventing compounds.

Adapted from S. Dresbach and A. Rossi, Ohio State University Extension Fact Sheet (Online). Available: http://ohioline.osu.edu/hyg-fact/5000/5050.html [August 1, 2006].

NUTRITION

People are vegetarians for different reasons—religious, political, social, economic, and health. As discussed earlier in the chapter, there are a number of types of vegetarians. People who subscribe to any of these vegetarian eating styles vary in age, gender, ethnicity, body weight, activity levels, and other characteristics. Regardless of type, vegetarians have nutritional needs based on their age, gender, activity level, and so on. Remember that all people, especially those who are active, must meet energy and nutritional needs for optimal performance and health.

General Vegetarian Concerns

Several nutrients present concern for people who consume a vegetarian diet. The ones of most concern are protein, iron, calcium, vitamin D, vitamin B_{12}, and zinc. These nutrients should be carefully monitored to ensure adequate consumption, especially in vegans, who consume the strictest vegetarian diet that includes no foods of animal origin. Fruititarians and those who consume macrobiotic diets have far more nutrient deficiencies than those just listed; thus, we will discuss them in this section because their diets are much too limited and they are, by definition, at risk for overall malnutrition.

Protein

People once thought that vegetarians had to consume "complete proteins" together in one meal. A food with complete protein is a one that has all *essential amino acids*—that is, all the amino acids that our bodies cannot produce from food and that we must therefore derive in their complete form from what we eat. Red meat, egg whites, and milk are examples of complete proteins. Most plant foods, however, do not contain complete proteins. Thus, vegetarians used to be told that they had to "complement" their proteins to obtain their complete proteins. So, for example, they had to consume rice and beans together to obtain all the amino acids found in red meat; consuming just rice without the beans would not do. Additional research conducted over the years found that complementary proteins do not need to be eaten at the same time, although they should be consumed in the same day to produce benefits. So, a person who eats rice for lunch should consume legumes in the evening to obtain his or her complete proteins for the day. This eating plan is important to ensure proper functioning of protein within the body.

The Recommended Dietary Allowance (RDA) for protein is 0.8 g per kg (0.36 g per lb) of body weight per day. Note that this is the RDA for a sedentary person who is free from disease. People who are more active require more protein, based on the type of activity. For example, on average, an active person who exercises about 30 minutes per day may require 1.0 to 1.1 g of protein per kg (0.45 to 0.5 g per lb) of body weight per day. However, a long-distance runner or other endurance athlete will need from 1.2 to 1.4 g of protein per kg (0.55 to 0.64 g per lb) of body weight per day. A novice competitive weightlifter will require about 1.4 to 1.6 g of protein per kg (0.64 to 0.73 g per lb) of body weight per day, but a more

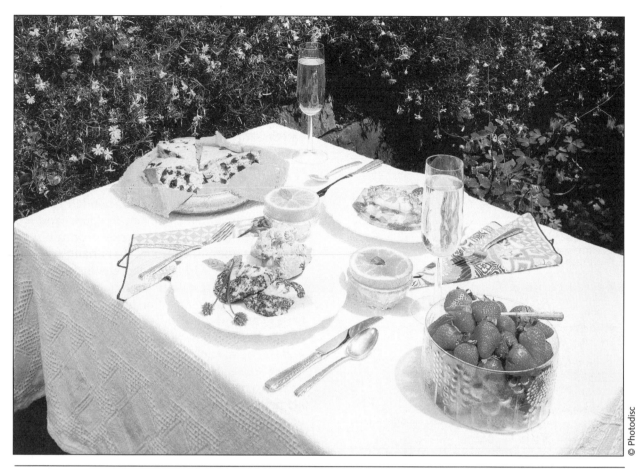

© Photodisc

The stereotype that vegetarian diets are boring is far from the truth. This vegetarian spread includes whole-grain scones with raisins, fresh grapefruit and strawberries, baked herbed soy patties, egg and soy-bacon omelet, and wine.

experienced weightlifter will need only 1.2 to 1.4 g of protein per kg (0.55 to 0.64 g per lb) of body weight per day. Because vegetarians, especially vegans, consume a large amount of plant protein, which is digested a bit differently than animal protein is, vegetarians are sometimes advised to consume 1.0 g of protein per kg (0.45 g per lb) of body weight per day. Thus, to obtain a crude estimate of protein needs, a vegetarian could just divide his or her body weight in pounds in half. The result would be the average amount of protein needed in grams per day. Varied plant sources can easily satisfy protein requirements. These include cooked beans, tofu, soy products, tempeh, seitan, nuts, seeds, and whole grains. For vegetarians who consume them, dairy products and eggs also provide protein. Of course, for semi-vegetarians and pesco-vegetarians, meat, poultry, and fish are sources of protein. See table 5.3 for the amount of protein in these foods.

Minerals

In general, vegetarians are able to meet their nutritional needs through diet alone, although doing so does take some planning. Occasionally (depending on the type of vegetarian), supplementation may be indicated. Because even standard grocery stores have many more options from which to choose than they did 10 years ago, vegetarians now have an easier time consuming nutritious, varied diets.

- **Iron.** Vegetarian diets are typically higher in total iron than nonvegetarian diets, but the iron in a vegetarian diet is not as bioavailable, that is, not as easily absorbed. Animal products like red meat contain heme iron, which is more bioavailable to the body than is the nonheme iron contained in plant products. For example, spinach contains a large amount of iron, but it is not absorbed as well as the iron in red meat is. This occurs because

Table 5.3 Vegetarian Food Sources of Protein

Food	Protein content (g)
Milk, skim, 1 cup (240 ml)	8
Yogurt, nonfat, 1 cup (113 g)	12
Egg, 1 medium (30 g)	6
Kidney beans, canned, 1/2 cup (55 g)	8
Tofu, 4 oz (120 g)	9
Soybeans, cooked, 1 cup (115 g)	29
Soy milk, plain, 1 cup (240 ml)	3 to 10
Soy yogurt, plain, 6 oz (180 g)	6
Tempeh, 1 cup (115 g)	31
Seitan, 4 oz (120 g)	15 to 31
Almonds, 1 oz (30 g)	6
Sunflower seeds, 1/4 cup (50 g)	6
Whole-wheat bread, 2 slices (160 g)	6
Peanut butter, 2 tbsp (30 g)	8

From S.L. Volpe, S.B. Sabelawski, and C.R. Mohr, 2007, *Fitness nutrition for special dietary needs* (Champaign, IL: Human Kinetics). Adapted from www.new-fitness.com/nutrition/protein.html and www.vrg.org/nutrition/protein.html.

compounds called ***phytates*** and oxalates bind to the iron to make it less available to the body. But vegetarians benefit from another effect. Because they consume more fruits, they have more vitamin C in their diets, which helps increase absorption of iron, especially iron from nonanimal products. Therefore, people who consume mostly nonheme iron should also consume foods rich in vitamin C, like orange juice, with their meals to enhance iron absorption (this is mostly a concern for those who have iron deficiency anemia). Coffee and tea decrease iron absorption because of the tannins that they contain. Tannin binds to iron to make it less available to the body. So, those who need to increase iron absorption should wait for an hour after consuming a meal to drink coffee or tea. If a person, vegetarian or nonvegetarian, becomes anemic because of iron deficiency, he or she must see a physician and a registered dietitian. Typically, high doses of iron supplementation are given until iron status is restored. See table 5.4 for vegetarian sources of iron.

- **Calcium**. The best bioavailable sources of calcium are dairy products. The vitamin D and calcium-to-protein ratio within these products are ideal for high absorption. For vegetarians who do not consume dairy products, good sources of calcium include dark leafy green vegetables (for example, kale and spinach), almonds, broccoli, calcium-fortified orange juice, tofu (fortified with calcium), soy milk (fortified with calcium), bok choy, and baked beans. Refer to chapter 4 and table 5.4 for other sources of calcium-rich foods. Because the calcium from these nondairy sources is less bioavailable than that in dairy products, people should consume these products with foods that contain vitamin D to enhance calcium absorption. In addition, decreasing salt intake while consuming calcium will help decrease urinary calcium excretion. Calcium supplementation is recommended for those who may not be able to achieve calcium recommendations. The type and timing of calcium supplements is important. Nonetheless, because of their high consumption of plant protein, most vegetarians have a less acidic environment in the kidneys compared with nonvegetarians; therefore, the kidneys retain more calcium. The better absorption is also a result of the body's ability to recognize that it needs more of a certain nutrient, especially when less is consumed. This favorable circumstance is not always the case because every person is different, so no one should strive to consume less of the recommended intake! Refer to chapter 4 for more information on the best types of calcium supplements and the best timing for them.

- **Zinc.** Zinc is involved in over 300 metabolic reactions in the body. Zinc is not readily absorbed in plant foods. Good vegetarian sources of zinc include sea vegetables, oats, seeds, greens, nutritional yeast, some whole grains, legumes, and fortified cereals. Refer to table 5.4 for the amount of zinc in these and other foods.

Vitamins

Like minerals, vitamins are important to health. Some vitamins, like some minerals, may be more affected than others are by vegetarian diets, especially diets that do not provide adequate variety.

- **Vitamin D**. This vitamin is not found naturally in many foods, but some foods are fortified with vitamin D. Vegans do not drink fortified cow's milk, but they can consume other foods fortified

Table 5.4 Vegetarian Food Sources of Problematic Minerals

Food	Mineral content (mg)
IRON	
Soybeans, cooked, 1 cup (115 g)	8.8
Blackstrap molasses, 2 tbsp (30 g)	7
Soy yogurt, plain, 6 oz (180 g)	1.4
Tempeh, 1 cup (115 g)	3.8
Lentils, cooked, 1 cup (115 g)	6.6
Kidney beans, cooked, 1 cup (115 g)	5.2
Black beans, cooked, 1 cup (115 g)	3.6
Bagel, enriched, 3 oz (90 g)	3.2
Spinach, cooked, 1 cup (115 g)	2.9
Raisins, 1/2 cup (60 g)	2.2
Brussels sprouts, cooked, 1 cup (115 g)	1.1
CALCIUM	
Soy milk or rice milk, 1 cup, calcium fortified (240 ml)	150 to 500
Collard greens, 1 cup (115 g)	304
Calcium-fortified orange juice, 8 oz (240 ml)	300
Soy yogurt, plain, 6 oz (180 g)	250
Bok choy, cooked, 1 cup (115 g)	158
Tempeh, 1 cup (115 g)	154
Mustard greens, cooked, 1 cup (115 g)	152
Almond butter, 2 tbsp (30 g)	86
Spinach, cooked, 1 cup (115 g)	2.9
ZINC	
Chickpeas, 7 oz (200 g)	2.8
Baked beans, 8 oz (225 g)	1.6
Vegetarian burger, 3.5 oz (100 g)	1.6
Pumpkin seeds, 20 g	1.3
Cheddar cheese, 1 oz (30 g)	1.2
Tahini paste (used to make hummus), 20 g	1.1

From S.L. Volpe, S.B. Sabelawski, and C.R. Mohr, 2007, *Fitness nutrition for special dietary needs* (Champaign, IL: Human Kinetics). Data from USDA Nutrient Database for Standard Reference, Release 12, 1998, and www.vegsoc.org/info/zinc.html.

with vitamin D, such as soy milk and cereals. Sun exposure is also a good way to obtain vitamin D. Nonetheless, people who live in the northern part of the United States, in New England, for example, do not have sufficient conversion of vitamin D on their skin from November through

February or March, because even on sunny days, the ultraviolet (UV) rays of the sun are too weak to make the conversion. Thus, if a person is not consuming enough vitamin D and lives in an area where conversion of vitamin D may be limited to certain times of the year, supplements may be recommended. This suggestion is especially important for vegans. Refer to table 5.5 for food sources of vitamin D.

Table 5.5   Vegetarian Food Sources of Problematic Vitamins

Food	Vitamin content
VITAMIN D[1]	
Milk, fortified, 1 cup (240 ml)	98
Margarine, 1 tbsp (15 g)	60
Dry cereal, 10% fortified, 3/4 cup (95 g)	40 to 50
Egg, 1 medium (vitamin D in the yolk) (30 g)	25
VITAMIN B$_{12}$[2]	
Fortified breakfast cereals, 100% fortified, 3/4 cup (95 g)	6.0
Fortified breakfast cereals, 25% fortified, 3/4 cup (95 g)	1.5
Yogurt, plain, skim, 1 cup (115 g)	1.4
Milk, 1 cup (240 ml)	0.9
1 egg, whole, hard boiled (30 g)	0.6
American pasteurized cheese food, 1 oz (30 g)	0.3

[1] In International Units (IU)

[2] In μg

From S.L. Volpe, S. B. Sabelawski, and C.R. Mohr, 2007, *Fitness nutrition for special dietary needs* (Champaign, IL: Human Kinetics). Data from www.healthlink.mcw.edu/article/982088787.html.

Supplement Resource

Though food is the best way to obtain nutrients, supplementation may be required for some vegetarians. Below is the Web site for the Office of Dietary Supplements (within the National Institutes of Health) that provides information on vitamin and mineral supplements.
http://dietary-supplements.info.nih.gov/

- **Vitamin B$_{12}$.** Vitamin B$_{12}$ is found in animal foods; plant foods contain little or no vitamin B$_{12}$. Vitamin B$_{12}$ is also found in dairy products and eggs but not in sufficient quantity to meet daily requirements. Some vegetarians (specifically vegans) have been shown to have low vitamin B$_{12}$ levels. Therefore, supplements or consumption of fortified foods is recommended. Older vegetarians, particularly older vegans, are advised to supplement because aging brings about a decrease in production of the protein called *intrinsic factor*, which is in the stomach and is necessary for absorption of vitamin B$_{12}$. Good food sources of vitamin B$_{12}$ include fortified breakfast cereals, fortified soy milk, nutritional yeast, and fortified meat analogs. Refer to table 5.5 for amounts of vitamin B$_{12}$ in these foods.

Nutrition for Active Vegetarians

The main concern for active vegetarians is to consume enough energy per day to maintain their energy expenditure. If they are doing this, they will usually meet their nutrient (vitamin and mineral) needs. If they are not, they should increase their consumption of foods that are good sources of nutrients referred to in the previous section or consider supplementation.

Well-controlled long-term studies assessing the effects of vegetarian diets on athletes have not been performed, but Barr and Rideout (2004) have made the following observations based on what has been conducted:

(1) Well-planned, appropriately supplemented vegetarian diets appear to effectively support athletic performance; (2) provided protein intakes are adequate to meet needs for total nitrogen and the essential amino acids, plant and animal protein sources appear to provide equivalent support to athletic training and performance; (3) vegetarians (particularly women) are at increased risk for non-anemic iron deficiency, which may limit endurance performance; (4) as a group, vegetarians have lower mean muscle creatine concentrations than do omnivores, and this may affect supra-maximal exercise performance. Because their initial muscle creatine concentrations are lower, vegetarians are likely to experience greater performance increments after creatine loading in activities that rely on the adenosine

triphosphate/phosphocreatine system; and (5) coaches and trainers should be aware that some athletes may adopt a vegetarian diet as a strategy for weight control. Accordingly, the possibility of a disordered eating pattern should be investigated if a vegetarian diet is accompanied by unwarranted weight loss.

Vegetarian athletes must plan their meals more carefully than athletes who are not vegetarians. Some general meal-planning recommendations for vegetarian athletes include the following:

- Choose a variety of foods including whole grains, fruits, legumes, nuts, seeds, and dairy products (if consumed).
- Choose whole, unrefined foods and limit intake of sweets, fats, and refined foods.
- Choose a variety of fruits and vegetables.

- Lacto-ovo vegetarians should choose low-fat dairy products.
- Vegans should include regular sources of vitamin D (if sun exposure is limited) and vitamin B$_{12}$.
- Consume adequate energy (kilocalories) and nutrients (vitamin and mineral).

The vegetarian food guide pyramid is an excellent guideline for vegans and other vegetarians (see figure 5.1).

The following meal plan is appropriate for most active vegetarians. You can modify the meal plan based on the type of vegetarian with whom you are working. For example, a lacto-ovo vegetarian could have cow's milk instead of soy milk, a pesco-vegetarian may want to replace tofu with salmon, and a vegan would replace honey with fruit spread. Again, the sample meal plans provided in this book are guidelines that will need to

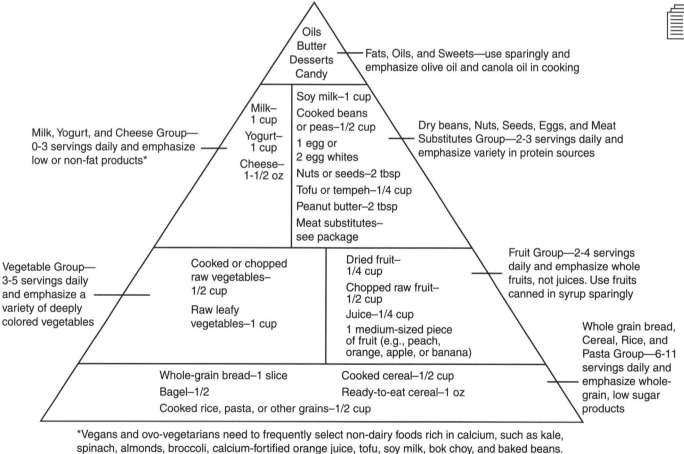

*Vegans and ovo-vegetarians need to frequently select non-dairy foods rich in calcium, such as kale, spinach, almonds, broccoli, calcium-fortified orange juice, tofu, soy milk, bok choy, and baked beans.

Figure 5.1   The vegetarian food guide pyramid.

From S.L. Volpe, S.B. Sabelawski, and C.R. Mohr, 2007, *Fitness nutrition for special dietary needs* (Champaign, IL: Human Kinetics).

Sample Meal Plan for Vegetarians

The sample meal plan provided in this chapter offers a variety of food choices, but it is not complete. The food choices shown here are meant to spark ideas for other meal plans. See tables A.1 through A.4 in the appendix for alternative food choices.

Breakfast

- 1 cup of bran flakes = 60 g
- 1 cup of fortified soy milk = 240 ml
- 1/4 cup of raisins = 57 g
- 1 medium banana = 130 g
- 1 cup of orange juice (calcium fortified) = 240 ml

Snack

- 1 slice of whole-wheat toast = 40 g
- 1 tbsp of peanut butter = 15 g
- 2 tsp of honey or 100% fruit spread = 10 g
- 12 oz of water = 360 ml

Lunch

- 1 cup of lentil soup = 240 ml
- 1 cup of mixed greens salad = 30 g
- 1 oz of sliced almonds = 28 g
- 1/4 cup of dried cranberries = 57 g
- 1/2 cup of mandarin oranges = 113 g
- 2 tbsp of salad dressing of choice = 30 g
- 1 whole-grain dinner roll = 80 g
- 1 tsp of margarine or butter = 5 g
- 1 cup of 100% juice = 240 ml

Snack

- 1 medium apple = 120 g
- 3 cups of microwave light popcorn = 90 g
- 8 oz of water = 240 ml

Dinner

- 1 cup of whole-wheat pasta with tomato sauce = 227 g
- 4 oz of tofu (calcium fortified) = 120 g
- 2 tbsp of parmesan cheese or soy cheese = 30 g
- 1 cup of cooked spinach = 220 g
- 1 cup of fresh fruit salad = 227 g
- 12 oz of water = 360 ml

Snack

- 1/2 whole-wheat bagel = 40 g
- 1 tbsp of almond butter = 15 g
- 1 cup of fortified soy milk = 240 ml

This sample meal plan provides at least 100% of the Dietary Reference Intakes (DRIs) for energy, protein, fiber, vitamins A, C, E, B_6, B_{12}, thiamin, riboflavin, niacin, folate, calcium, iron, magnesium, phosphorus, zinc, and approximately

- 2,500 kcal (10,450 kJ),
- 94 g of protein,
- 84 g of fat,
- 65 g of fiber, and
- 3,900 mg of sodium.

From S.L. Volpe, S.B. Sabelawski, and C.R. Mohr, 2007, *Fitness nutrition for special dietary needs* (Champaign, IL: Human Kinetics).

---

be customized for each person, based on factors such as activity level, gender, body weight, and likes and dislikes.

PHYSICAL ACTIVITY

Unlike other special populations discussed in this book, vegetarians are offered no specific exercise recommendations. That vegetarianism is not an impediment for athletes is clearly shown by the number of vegetarian athletes who have won national championships, Olympic medals,

and other accolades in various sports. Here is a sampling of famous vegetarian athletes:

- Al Beckles (bodybuilder)
- Sorya Bonali (Olympic ice skater)
- Les Brown (veteran runner)
- Peter Burwash (tennis)
- Andreas Cahling (bodybuilder)
- Chris Campbell (1980 world champion wrestler)
- Joanna Conway (ice skater)

- Sylvia Cranston (triathlete)
- Di Edwards (runner, Olympic semifinalist)
- Katie Fitzgibbon (marathon runner)
- Clare Francis (sailor)
- Louis Freitas (bodybuilder)
- Carol Gould (marathon runner)
- Sammy Green (runner)
- Sally Hibberd (British women's mountain bike champion)
- Sharon Hounsell (Miss Wales bodybuilding champion)
- Roger Hughes (Welsh national ski champion)
- Kathy Johnson (Olympic gymnast)
- Alan Jones (British ski jumper)
- Jack LaLanne (fitness guru)
- Silken Laumann (Olympic rower)
- Judy Leden (British, European, and world hang-gliding champion)
- Jack Maitland (triathlete)
- Leslie Marx (fencer, 1996 woman's epee national champion)
- Kirsty McDermott (runner)
- Lindford McFarquar (bodybuilder)
- Robert Millar (cyclist)
- Edwin Moses (Olympic runner, gold medalist)
- Martina Navratilova (tennis champion)
- Dave Scott (five-time winner of the Ironman Triathlon)
- Lucy Stephens (triathlete)
- Kirsty Wade (runner)

The list is adapted from www.veggie.org/veggie/famous.veg.athletes. shtml.

The more intense the exercise regimen in which a vegetarian is partaking, the more important it is for that person to consume an adequate amount of energy and nutrients.

A person who is just beginning an exercise program should see his or her physician and work with an exercise physiologist (if one is available) to map out an appropriate exercise program.

The FITT principle (frequency, intensity, time, type of exercise) should be considered as well. In general, a person should exercise on most days of the week, at about 60% to 80% of his or her predicted maximal heart rate (predicted maximal heart rate = 220 – age [Karvonen method]; multiplying this number by 0.60 and 0.80 gives a range within 60% to 80% of predicted maximal heart rate; higher ranges can be used, depending on goals) for about 30 minutes (either all at once or accumulated throughout the day). The person should perform activities that he or she enjoys (preferably varied throughout the week, but walking is simple and easy to do). Depending on individual goals, the person can perform at higher intensity, for longer duration, and more frequently. Resistance training is always recommended for a minimum of 2 days per week. Yoga and Pilates, both excellent methods of training for all ages and exercise goals, are other ways to increase strength. Performing yoga and Pilates, or a combination of the two, 2 to 3 days per week, in addition to performing an aerobic activity on most days of the week, will lead to gains in aerobic fitness and strength.

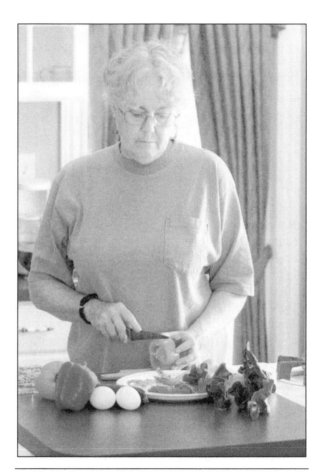

By including protein sources, whole-grain foods, and a wide variety of deep and brightly colored vegetables, vegetarians can achieve nutrition, which will support good overall health as well as a beneficial dose of physical activity.

Myths About Vegetarian Athletes

People often ask whether they will be able to perform as well in their respective athletic events if they become vegetarians. The answer is yes, but . . . . The *but* is not because a vegetarian diet cannot sustain the high levels of energy expenditure resulting from intense, long-duration exercise; it stems from the fact that eating well, whether a person is a vegetarian or not, is crucial to overall exercise performance, as we have stated throughout the book. Therefore, the first thing that you need to make clear to an athlete or exerciser who wants to become a vegetarian is that eating healthy and consuming enough energy are still important. Several athletes have come to us and said, "I have become a vegetarian so that I can eat more ice cream and french fries." Although people can have personal reasons for becoming vegetarians, that reason is not a suitable one, nor will the resulting diet produce better performance or health! So, can a person be a strong athlete or exerciser and be a vegetarian? Yes, with healthy eating and by eating enough!

CASE STUDY

In this case study, our guest dietitian reports on an adolescent athlete who became a vegetarian but because of poor choices was becoming tired and performing poorly. But with the help of our guest dietitian, the young athlete was able to improve her food consumption while remaining a vegetarian and improve her performance.

Jenna is a 16-year-old soccer goalkeeper. She is an all-state player on her high school team and plays for an elite club team as well. At 68 in. (172 cm) and 129 lb (59 kg), Jenna is undersized for her position. She hopes to play for the United States national team and definitely for a Division I college program in upcoming years. Jenna's strength as a goalkeeper comes from her speed and athleticism. Coaches have recommended that Jenna increase her size and strength to avoid being knocked around in the box. Jenna has an excellent body image and is willing to gain weight, but not at the expense of losing speed. Because some of her peers have complained of sluggishness when they gained weight, Jenna is particularly wary

about this happening to her. She would like to weigh between 145 and 150 lb (between 66 and 68 kg). Her goal is to increase lean body mass while lowering her body fat, currently estimated at 20.5% by skinfold assessment.

Jenna and her best friend decided to become vegetarians for ethical reasons on their 16th birthdays (7 months ago for Jenna). She eats no meat, poultry, fish, or dairy products but will eat eggs. Jenna's mother has been concerned that her daughter is not meeting her nutritional needs, so Jenna agreed to work with a registered dietitian when her energy level started to become consistently low. She feels tired and sluggish in workouts, becomes drowsy during school (but cannot sleep at night), and has stopped gaining strength in the weight room. A recent medical examination by the pediatrician revealed iron depletion (low serum **ferritin** levels), but not iron deficiency anemia (low **hematocrit** and **hemoglobin** levels). Her serum ferritin level is 7 (normal range is 20 to 120 µg per ml), her hemoglobin level is 13 (normal range is 12 to 16 g per dl), and her hematocrit is 47% (normal range is 37% to 47%). The pediatrician found no other causes of her symptoms. It would be beneficial to determine whether these hemoglobin and hematocrit levels reveal true iron depletion or relative iron depletion from increased plasma volume because of her high levels of physical activity, but no laboratory analyses on her blood had previously been conducted. The physician prescribed a chewable multivitamin with iron, but Jenna had not been taking it because she did not like the taste. Jenna reports normal menstrual periods.

Jenna is a fussy eater whose diet includes little variety. She reports that her daily intake typically consists of a bagel, cream cheese, and hot tea for breakfast; nothing for lunch except a cola; and either french fries or vegetarian hot dogs with chocolate soy milk for dinner. She admits to being bored with her diet and being hungry and lethargic almost all day long. She always goes to bed hungry. She used to eat a large bowl of ice cream right before bed but discontinued that routine when she became a vegetarian. She has tried the tofu and soy ice creams available but does not like them. She likes grains, eggs, fruits, beans, and many of the vegetarian products from the frozen food section. She especially likes Mexican and Italian foods. Except for potatoes and spinach salads, Jenna states that she hates all vegetables.

Overall, Jenna and her mother agree that the goals of our sessions are to improve energy levels, increase iron intake, and gain weight and strength. Jenna is determined and compliant and has been ready to add new challenges at each meeting; other clients have progressed much more slowly.

Meeting 1: Improve iron status

Teaching point: Iron has a critical role in aerobic function and overall health. Because Jenna had documented iron depletion, had symptoms of iron deficiency anemia, and was clearly eating inadequate iron, our first goal was to work on this shortfall. Our overall goal was for Jenna to consume 20 to 25 mg of iron per day, and I emphasized the importance of using an iron supplement as well.

Here is what we did:

- Changed the chewable vitamin to a tablet multivitamin with iron along with a 50 mg elemental iron tablet. Jenna took these each night with orange juice (for increased iron absorption by means of the vitamin C in the orange juice).

- Changed breakfast from a bagel to either a large bowl of iron-fortified cereal (we found three that Jenna enjoys) with soy milk or two slices of iron-fortified bread with two fried eggs, soy cheese, and a glass of orange juice. Many nights she made the egg sandwich before going to bed and just heated it in the microwave in the morning. She stopped having tea along with breakfast because the tea could be decreasing iron absorption (tannins in tea bind with iron to decrease its absorption).

- Started packing lunch. Jenna agreed to canned bean soup; a trail mix of nuts, raisins, and chocolate; and soy yogurt. I explained that this lunch had 12 mg of iron and that she previously was consuming 0 mg of iron at lunch.

- Took advantage of her fondness for spinach salads. Jenna has one every night at dinner with strawberries or mandarin oranges for vitamin C to increase iron absorption from the spinach.

- Sometimes added a large bowl of sweetened iron-fortified cereal before bed, which she enjoyed because she had missed having ice cream.

Meeting 2: Increase meal frequency

Teaching point: Although Jenna was now eating 2,400 kcal per day (10,032 kJ per day), a substantial improvement over her initial 1,600 kcal per day (6,688 kJ pcr day), she was still well short of meeting her energy requirement of about 3,100 kcal per day. Adding meals and snacks would be the critical tool for increasing energy to our goal of 3,500 kcal per day (14,630 kJ per day) to support a gain in lean mass.

Here is what we did:

- Created a meal plan that structured breakfast, lunch, dinner, a packed after-school snack, and a bedtime snack.

- Because breakfast, lunch, and dinner were now habits, our primary focus was the snacks. We came up with three 500 kcal (2,090 kJ) after-school snacks that would not bother her at practice (for example, sports bar, fruit juice box, banana, peanut butter and jelly on whole-wheat bread, soy yogurt-covered raisins, Gatorade). She had already agreed to have the cereal and soy milk before bed each night.

- Created a grocery list that Jenna could give to her mother so that Jenna would have the ingredients and foods that she needed for packing and home eating.

Meeting 3: Meet protein needs

Teaching point: Many vegetarian athletes struggle to meet protein needs. Jenna had proved to be no exception, at least initially. We set her protein goal at 100 g of protein per day because of her goal to increase lean mass. At the time of this meeting she was consuming about 60 to 70 g of protein per day. I provided Jenna with a resource list of the protein content of vegetarian foods.

Here's what we did:

- Added a sports bar for Jenna to eat on the bus on the way to school (added 15 g of protein). We selected this time period because breakfast had not been satiating her.

- Added garbanzo beans or sunflower seeds and shredded soy cheese to spinach salads.

- Started using a high-protein version of soy milk for cereal.

- Added tofu or flavored soy powder to smoothies.

Meeting 4: Improve Variety

Teaching point: Because Jenna was still eating almost exactly the same foods every day, I included the goal of improving the variety of her food consumption. I believed that adding variety would help Jenna consistently attain all the nutrients that she needs and improve palatability. I also thought that adding different foods would give Jenna a great opportunity to learn cooking skills.

Here's what we did:

- We had our 1-hour consultation in Jenna's family kitchen.
- I gave her a binder to collect our recipes and ideas.
- During the first session, Jenna learned to cook three different dinners: tofu crumble chili, black bean enchiladas (because she likes Mexican food), and vegetarian lasagna (because she likes Italian food).

Future Sessions

Future sessions will include follow-up on previous goals, more cooking sessions, body composition analysis, and opportunity for questions. I have asked Jenna's mother to take her back to the pediatrician for a repeat blood test in 2 months (which will be 4 months after her first test).

Jenna has just finished her soccer season, so I am unable to assess any performance changes based on our work together, but Jenna does report a much improved energy level. She also reported that her weight-room maximum lifts have increased about 30% in 2 months, and she has gained 9 lb (4.1 kg) in 2 months. Her mother says that she is in a much better mood, as well!

Michelle S. Rockwell, MS, RD
Sports Nutrition Consultant
Durham, North Carolina

Overweight and Obesity

Overweight and obesity are associated with the onset of significant health problems. Both have risen to epidemic levels in the Western hemisphere over the past few decades and are increasing at alarming rates worldwide (Ogden et al., 2006; Hedley et al., 2004).

OVERWEIGHT, OBESITY, AND HEALTH

The obesity epidemic is of concern because both overweight and obesity are precursors to numerous major health problems including, but not limited to, cardiovascular disease, type 2 diabetes mellitus, hypertension, sleep apnea, dyslipidemia, *osteoarthritis*, and several types of cancer (Kopelman, 2000) (table 6.1). Therefore, we need to examine nutritional, behavioral, and exercise paradigms that assist in the treatment of overweight and obesity.

Classifying Overweight and Obesity

Several methods can be used to assess healthy versus unhealthy weight:

- **Weight charts that classify people as healthy weight, overweight, or obese.** These charts rely on a simple correlation of height and weight. The advantage of these charts is that they are easy to use, requiring no technology. The disadvantage is that they are not precise because they rely on generalizations, and not everyone falls into a generalizeable category. The charts do not take into account bone mineral density or lean body mass. Thus, a person who is muscular or has dense bones may be classified as obese, when in fact he or she has little body fat. For the general population, this issue typically does not apply, but it does apply to athletes, for whom the charts can be inaccurate. Table 6.2 is an example of such a chart. To convert feet to meters multiply the number of feet by .305; to convert pounds to kg multiply the number of pounds by .454.

- **Weight can also be classified according to body mass index (BMI) (table 6.3).** BMI is calculated as weight in kilograms divided by height in meters squared, providing a useful estimate of the level of obesity. Another way to calculate BMI is by taking weight in pounds, dividing the result by height in inches squared, and then multiplying that number by 702. A person who has a BMI of

Table 6.1   Frequent Comorbidities of Obesity

Greatly increased	Moderately increased	Slightly increased
Diabetes	Coronary heart disease	Cancer—breast in postmenopausal women, endometrial, colon
Gallbladder disease	Hypertension	Reproductive hormone abnormalities
Dyslipidemia	Osteoarthritis (knees)	Polycystic ovary syndrome
Insulin resistance	Hyperuricemia and gout	Impaired fertility
Breathlessness		Low back pain due to obesity
Sleep apnea		Increased anesthetic risk
		Fetal defects associated with maternal obesity

Adapted from World Health Organization (WHO) 1997, *Obesity: Preventing and managing the global epidemic—Report of a WHO Consultation on Obesity.*

Table 6.2   Body-Weight Classifications

Height (in.)	Weight (in lb)																
58	91	96	100	105	110	115	119	124	129	134	138	143	148	153	158	162	167
59	94	99	104	109	114	119	124	128	133	138	143	148	153	158	163	168	173
60	97	102	107	112	118	123	128	133	138	143	148	153	158	163	168	174	179
61	100	106	111	116	122	127	132	137	143	148	153	158	164	169	174	180	185
62	104	109	115	120	126	131	136	142	147	153	158	164	169	175	180	186	191
63	107	113	118	124	130	135	141	146	152	158	163	169	175	180	186	191	197
64	110	116	122	128	134	140	145	151	157	163	169	174	180	186	192	197	204
65	114	120	126	132	138	144	150	156	162	168	174	180	186	192	198	204	210
66	118	124	130	136	142	148	155	161	167	173	179	186	192	198	204	210	216
67	121	127	134	140	146	153	159	166	172	178	185	191	198	204	211	217	223
68	125	131	138	144	151	158	164	171	177	184	190	197	203	210	216	223	230
69	128	135	142	149	155	162	169	176	182	189	196	203	209	216	223	230	236
70	132	139	146	153	160	167	174	181	188	195	202	209	216	222	229	236	243
71	136	143	150	157	165	172	179	186	193	200	208	215	222	229	236	243	250
72	140	147	154	162	169	177	184	191	199	206	213	221	228	235	242	250	258
73	144	151	159	166	174	182	189	197	204	212	219	227	235	242	250	257	265
74	148	155	163	171	179	186	194	202	210	218	225	233	241	249	256	264	272
75	152	160	168	176	184	192	200	208	216	224	232	240	248	256	264	272	279
BMI	19	20	21	22	23	24	25	26	27	28	29	30	31	32	33	34	35
	Healthy weight						Overweight					Obese					

Adapted from the National Heart, Lung, and Blood Institute (NHLBI), a division of the National Institutes of Health. www.nhlbi.nih.gov.

18.5 to 24.9 is considered to have a healthy body weight. Overweight is defined as having a BMI of 25.0 to 29.9. Anything above that is considered obese. Table 6.3 provides a more precise body-weight classification by BMI, along with the risk of comorbidities associated with each. BMI is a valuable baseline assessment tool for the general population, but it is just one of many factors necessary to make a true diagnosis of overweight and obesity. For example, lean body mass is not taken into account in the calculation of BMI. Therefore, some people classified as overweight or obese are really rather lean. These people may be overweight, but they are not overfat. Thus, the same caution needs to be taken with BMI as previously discussed with body-weight charts. Although BMI is easy to calculate and is a relatively good measure of overweight or obesity in the general population, athletic individuals who are muscular or who have dense bones may be miscategorized using BMI.

• **Assessing body composition,** that is, measuring the fat-versus-muscle composition of a person, is the most accurate method to evaluate whether a person is overfat. As discussed earlier, a person can be overweight but not overfat. Several methods can be used to evaluate body composition, including skinfold calipers, bioelectrical impedance analysis (BIA), air-displacement plethysmography, underwater weighing (or hydrodensitometry), and dual-energy X-ray absorptiometry (DEXA). Here are descriptions of each:

- The **skinfold method** estimates total body fat from measures of subcutaneous fat that are obtained with calipers that pinch the fat at specified anatomical locations. A number of different measurement sites can be used, and a variety of formulas are used with skinfold calipers. From one to seven sites can be assessed. Typically, the larger the number of sites assessed, the more accurate the measurement is. Let the client know that skinfold measurements can be in error by as much as 10%. The recommended approach is simply to state the total sum of skinfolds and assess how that changes over time, rather than to calculate percent body fat. Most people, however, want to know a percentage. One major benefit is that calipers are portable, convenient, and affordable.

- **Bioelectrical impedance analysis** (BIA) passes a low-level electrical signal through the body. This method relies on the fact that lean tissue and water conduct electricity better than fat does. The amount of resistance to the signal determines total body water. The value is then used to estimate percentage of body fat. The several types of BIAs are generally simple to use and reasonably reliable in the general population, except in people who have large changes in extracellular fluids (for example, renal patients). BIA has about a 5% coefficient of variation (error rate).

- **Underwater weighing (hydrodensitometry)** is considered one of the gold standards of body-composition assessment. Hydrodensitometry assumes that the body is composed of fat mass and fat-free mass. The calculations are formulated from this

Table 6.3   Body Mass Index (BMI) and Risk of Comorbidities

Classification	BMI (kg/m²)	Risk of comorbidities
Underweight	<18.5	Low (but risk of other clinical problems increased)
Normal range	18.5 to 24.9	Average
Overweight	25.0 to 29.9	Increased
Obese class I	30.0 to 34.9	Moderate
Obese class II	35.0 to 39.9	Severe
Obese class III	≥40.0	Very severe

Adapted from the National Heart, Lung, and Blood Institute (NHLBI), a division of the National Institutes of Health. www.nhlbi.nih.gov.

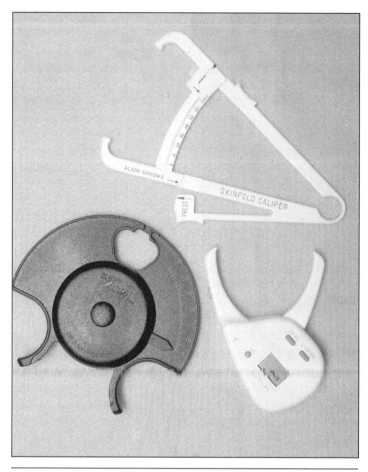

A variety of affordable and effective skinfold calipers are available.

assumption. This technique is more technical and requires a higher level of training than most others do. Hydrodensitometry also requires more equipment: a large tank with water, a chair with a measuring scale, and weights to keep a person submerged. Although this method is reliable and precise, it may underestimate body fat in extremely muscular people and overestimate body fat in children and elderly people (because of periods of rapid bone growth and rapid bone resorption, respectively). The coefficient of variation for hydrodensitometry is about 5%.

- **Air-displacement plethysmography** (Bod Pod for adults or Pea Pod for children) is a relatively new method of estimating body composition. Air-displacement plethysmography is similar to hydrodensitometry, but the subject, instead of displacing water through submersion, enters the pod and displaces air within it after the device is sealed. This method is reliable, but the pods, of course, are not as convenient or portable as skinfold calipers or BIA. Air-displacement plethysmography has an error rate of about 5%.

The number of overweight people in the United States has increased substantially, to more than 65% of adults (Hedley et al., 2004; Ogden et al., 2006). Worldwide, over 1 billion adults are considered overweight and 300 million are obese. In 2003 to 2004, 32.2% of the United States population was considered obese, defined as a BMI of greater than 30.0 (Ogden et al.). Although the incidence of overweight and obesity in other countries is not necessarily growing as fast as it is in the United States, the proportions have increased over the years, even in countries with traditionally low rates of overweight and obesity, such as France and Norway. Table 6.4 provides some international statistics on the percentage of adult males and females who are obese.

Additional Factors in Weight and Health

Another important determination of the risks associated with overweight and obesity is body-weight distribution. Traditionally, the two body types used in assessments are android (central or abdominal) obesity and gynoid (lower body or hip) obesity (figure 6.1). Android and gynoid obesity are determined through a simple waist-to-hip ratio. A waist-to-hip ratio greater than 0.80 in women or greater than 0.95 in men indicates increased risk of disease. Davi et al. (2002) reported that people who carry their weight more centrally (android) are at greater risk for coronary heart disease and diabetes mellitus than are people who carry their weight in the lower body (hip region).

Being thinner does not always mean being healthier. A landmark study published in 1989 noted that people who are overweight but physically active on a regular basis have a lower risk of mortality than those who are of normal weight but are not physically fit (Blair et al., 1989). Therefore, weight status and health are not always synonymous. Furthermore, a person who is overweight but not overfat is healthier than a person who is of normal weight or underweight but has a high percentage of body fat. We cannot judge a book by its cover. More often than not, however, overweight and obese people are not physically active, so exercise and nutrition intervention will be required to improve body weight and thus health.

Table 6.4 Percentage of Obese Adults in Countries Around the World

Country	Percentage of adult males (age 15 and older, unless otherwise specified) classified as obese	Percentage of adult females (age 15 and older, unless otherwise specified) classified as obese
Norway	7%	6%
Netherlands	10%	11%
Spain	13%	11%
Kuwait[1]	36.7%	38.2%
Ireland	14%	11%
Bosnia	16%	25%
Finland	21%	22%
Paraguay[2]	20%	36%
Tunisia	22.7%	6.7%
Morocco[3]	18%	5.7%
East Asia (China, Korea, Taiwan)[4]	38%	51%
South Asia (India and Pakistan)[4]	58%	75%

[1]From Al-Kandari, Y. (2006). Data are for those age 20 and older. www.ncbi.nlm.nih.gov/entrez/query.fcgi?cmd=Retrieve&db=PubMed&dopt=Citation&list_uids=16629871.

[2]From Filozof, Gonzalez, Sereday, Mazza, and Braguinsky (2001).

[3] Mokhtar, N., Elati, J., Chabir, R., Bour, A., Elkari, K., Schlossman, N.P., Caballero, B., and Aguenaou, H. Diet culture and obesity in northern Africa. J Nutrition (2001). 131:887S-892S. www.ncbi.nlm.nih.gov/entrez/query.fcgi?cmd=Retrieve&db=PubMed&dopt=Citation&list_uids=11238780.

[4]Values based on waist circumference >90 cm for men and >80 cm for women in Asia. www.medscape.com/viewarticle/544229.

Unless otherwise noted, data from www.euro.who.int/obesity. Retrieved July 16, 2006.

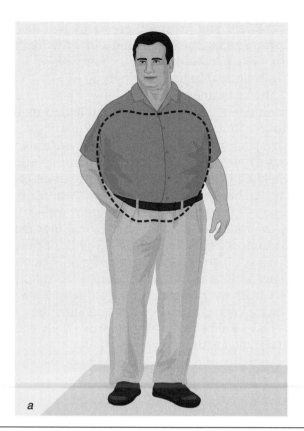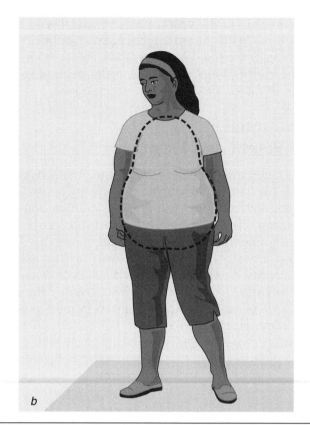

Figure 6.1 *(a)* Android obesity, also referred to as apple-shaped obesity; *(b)* gynoid obesity, also referred to as pear-shaped obesity. Android obesity presents greater risk of coronary heart disease, hypertension, stroke, high blood lipids, and type 2 diabetes.

Reprinted, by permission, from J.H. Wilmore and D.L. Costill, 2003, *Physiology of sport and exercise,* 3rd ed. (Champaign, IL: Human Kinetics), 679.

BASICS OF WEIGHT MANAGEMENT

Hundreds of different fad diets, gadgets, and weight-loss supplements are available. Those who have patented these items are thriving monetarily from the obesity epidemic. In reality, experts agree that the only way to reduce body weight safely is through moderate energy restriction and increased physical activity to change the energy balance equation (Jakicic et al., 2001). Weight loss requires a person to be in negative energy balance, whereas weight gain and weight maintenance require an energy surplus or energy balance, respectively. Thus, the two main factors that must be calculated and managed are how much energy is being expended and how much energy is being consumed.

Components of Energy Expenditure

Total energy expenditure (TEE) includes essentially four components (figure 6.2):

- Basal metabolic rate (BMR), also known as basal energy expenditure (BEE); resting metabolic rate (RMR), also known as resting energy expenditure (REE)
- Diet-induced *thermogenesis* (DIT), also known as thermic effect of food (TEF)
- Thermic effect of activity
- Nonexercise activity thermogenesis (NEAT)

- BMR (or BEE) and RMR (or REE) are often used interchangeably, although differences exist.

Although the values are often estimated for convenience, they are more accurately measured when an individual is in a rested state by ***indirect calorimetry***. For both BMR and RMR the person is required to be in a fasted state for at least 8 hours, but the BMR measurement is more accurate because the person does not have to travel to the site to have his or her BMR assessed (in a hospital or a metabolic ward, for example). The traveling would increase metabolic rate simply because of the extra movement involved (walking to the car, walking into the building for the measurement, and so on). RMR is commonly used in research, but because many subjects must travel to the study site to be assessed, it is typically about 5% greater than BMR. BMR is defined as the energy required for life support (for example, respiration and circulation), so no external factors play a role in this value. BMR accounts for approximately 60% to 75% of total energy expenditure (Danforth, 1985). BMR is affected by the ratio of overall body mass (bone, muscle, organ tissue) to the less active components (adipose tissue). Because muscle is more metabolically active than adipose tissue is, its contribution to overall BMR is greater. Therefore, the standard recommendation is for people to modify their diet and exercise regimens to decrease the loss of muscle tissue, which often accompanies weight loss, besides increasing their energy expenditure through exercise.

• Dietary induced thermogenesis (DIT), or the thermic effect of food, is the energy required for digestion and absorption of food. DIT makes up 5% to 15% of total energy expenditure (Daly et al., 1985). This number is not constant; it changes based on the composition of the diet. For example, a mixed diet provides a greater increase in DIT than a diet that is high in carbohydrate. Remember, however, that the overall contribution of DIT to energy expenditure is limited, so even drastic dietary changes (such as a diet high in protein, which causes the largest increase in DIT) will not significantly affect DIT or, subsequently, total energy expenditure.

• The thermic effect of activity is the most variable component of total energy expenditure. In general, activity accounts for approximately 20% to 40% of total energy expenditure, but studies have demonstrated that this percentage can

be higher in extremely active people or lower in extremely sedentary people (Horton, 1983; Ravussin & Bogardus, 1992). The intensity, type, duration, and frequency of the activity will alter this percentage, even if these change daily. The important concept to teach your clients is that they must maintain physical activity on a regular basis.

• Another important aspect to total energy expenditure is nonexercise activity thermogenesis (NEAT). NEAT has been defined in different ways, but it is often defined as the collective energy expended through various activities of daily living—the energy expended through activities such as fidgeting, standing versus sitting, spontaneous activity, and so on (Kotz & Levine, 2005; Novak, Zhang, & Levine, 2006). NEAT is significantly variable among individuals. Levine et al. (2005) reported that obese people expend less energy through NEAT than do people of healthy weight, even after the obese people lost weight. According to Kotz and Levine (2005), "Mounting evidence suggests that NEAT is critical in determining a person's susceptibility to body fat deposition and is a major factor in human obesity." People who adopt NEAT-enhanced behaviors can

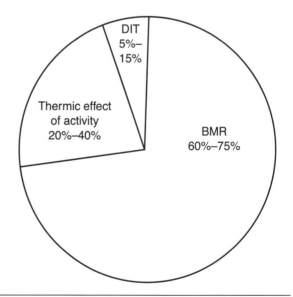

Figure 6.2 This pie chart depicts, on average, the percentages provided by each component of total energy expenditure. Note that basal metabolic rate makes up the greatest amount of total energy expenditure.

expend about 350 kcal per day above their usual energy expenditure (Levine et al.).

Calculating Energy Needs

A number of factors play a role in weight gain, weight maintenance, or weight loss. Very simply, weight loss occurs when energy output exceeds energy intake. The energy equivalent of 1 lb (0.45 kg) of body fat is 3,500 kcal (14,630 kJ); therefore, a deficit of 3,500 kcal is necessary for a 1 lb weight loss. Ideally, this weight loss would be made up completely of fat, but losing fat mass without losing some muscle mass along with it is difficult. Normally, weight loss consists largely of fat loss, especially if the weight loss occurs through a combination of exercise (including some resistance training) and a deficit in energy intake.

Health experts generally recommend a weight loss of 0.5 to 2.0 lb (about 0.5 to 1.0 kg) per week, which would require a deficit of 250 to 1,000 kcal (1,045 to 4,180 kJ) per day. The person should achieve this deficit through both a reduction in energy intake and an increase in energy expenditure. Rapid weight loss can be dangerous and increases the risk of weight regain (Perri, 1998). Furthermore, rapid weight loss represents a loss of fluid and lean body mass instead of actual fat loss. The modest energy reduction discussed earlier will allow slower but continual weight loss. This approach can be frustrating for people who want to lose weight, because they have heard about fad diets that hold out promises like "lose 15 lb (6.8 kg) in just 10 weeks." Many people therefore believe that quick weight loss should be their goal. When clients come to you with that hope, remind them that they did not gain all that weight in 10 weeks, so it would be unrealistic to lose it in that short a time.

There are many ways to determine energy requirements. As previously discussed, indirect calorimetry, which can assess BMR, DIT, and thermic effect of activity, is one of the most accurate methods of measuring energy expenditure, although it is not practical for clinicians to perform that kind of assessment on a day-to-day basis. But a number of validated methods can be used to estimate total energy expenditure. Although clinicians most often use the Harris–Benedict equation to estimate energy needs, other prediction equations exist as well (Daly et al., 1985; Mifflin et al., 1990). Another commonly used equation is the Mifflin–St. Jeor equation, which predicts resting energy expenditure (REE) in men and women (Mifflin et al.).

All these equations are based on body height, body weight, and gender, because all three characteristics affect resting energy expenditure. Although these equations have been validated, they have limitations because they are not direct measurements. Recent literature has suggested that predicted values for BMR are often higher than actual expenditure in specific populations, like those who are obese, so they should be used with caution with obese individuals. Frankenfield, Roth-Yousey, and Compher (2005) published a systematic review to evaluate the accuracy of predictive equations for resting metabolic rate in nonobese and obese people, and in people of various ethnic groups and age groups. These researchers classified the following four prediction equations as the most frequently used in clinical practice: Harris–Benedict, Mifflin–St. Jeor, Owen, and the World Health Organization–Food and Agriculture Organization–United Nations University (WHO–FAO–UNU). Frankenfield et al. (2005) reported that the Mifflin–St. Jeor equation was the most reliable of all the equations. It predicted RMR within 10% in both nonobese and obese people and had the tightest error range. The researchers stated, however, that older adults and ethnic minorities living in the United States were underrepresented in the development and validation of prediction equations. They emphasized that clinicians should consider using indirect calorimetry if possible, particularly if the prediction equations fail the patient in any way.

For an explanation of how to use the Mifflin–St. Jeor and Harris–Benedict equations to estimate energy requirements, see *"Using Equations to Predict Energy Requirements"* (page 95).

NUTRITION

Any sound weight-loss program includes behavioral treatment, physical activity, and nutrition modification. Nutrition modification must include a moderate reduction in energy intake and a focus on the quality of the foods consumed. When a sound nutrition program is combined with a good exercise and behavioral program, significant weight loss will ensue.

Using Equations to Predict Energy Requirements

After BMR is calculated from either indirect calorimetry or with a prediction equation, DIT and the thermic effect of activity must be calculated. If there is time to assess DIT and the thermic effect of activity directly by indirect calorimetry, that would be the best method. Realistically, however, the prediction equation to calculate BMR is often used, and from that point DIT and the thermic effect of activity can be estimated. On average, 10% of BMR is used to estimate DIT. Then, depending on the person's activity level, a range of about 20% to 40% is typically used to estimate the thermic effect of activity. With athletes, however, this can go as high as 75%. The thermic effect of activity must be assessed based on frequency, duration, and intensity of exercise (see the following activity factors).

To calculate a person's total energy expenditure, begin with a prediction equation to obtain BMR. The Mifflin–St. Jeor equation is recommended. The Mifflin–St. Jeor equation (Mifflin et al., 1990) for males and females follows:

$$\text{Male: BMR} = (10 \times \text{weight}) + (6.25 \times \text{height}) - (5 \times \text{age}) + 5$$

$$\text{Female: BMR} = (10 \times \text{weight}) + (6.25 \times \text{height}) - (5 \times \text{age}) - 161$$

The Harris–Benedict equation (Harris & Benedict, 1919) is frequently used as well:

$$\text{Male: BMR} = 66.47 + (13.75 \times \text{weight}) + (5 \times \text{height}) - (6.76 \times \text{age})$$

$$\text{Female: BMR} = 655.1 + (9.56 \times \text{weight}) + (1.85 \times \text{height}) - (4.68 \times \text{age})$$

Remember that these equations require weight in kilograms (pounds divided by 2.2 = kilograms), height in centimeters (inches multiplied by 2.54 = centimeters), and age in years.

To calculate total energy expenditure, the BMR has to be multiplied by the proper activity factor:

- 1.200 = sedentary (little or no exercise)
- 1.375 = lightly active (light exercise or sports 1 to 3 days per week)
- 1.550 = moderately active (moderate exercise or sports 3 to 5 days per week)
- 1.725 = very active (hard exercise or sports 6 to 7 days per week)
- 1.900 = extra active (very hard exercise or sports and physical job)

From: www.scientificpsychic.com/health/cron1.html.

Thus, first calculate BMR based on a prediction equation and then multiply that value by 10% to obtain DIT. Then, multiply the BMR by one of the activity factors to obtain the thermic effect of activity. Finally, add all three numbers together to obtain total energy expenditure (if using the activity factor, there is no need to add it back to the BMR because the "1" in front of the activity factor will calculate the energy expenditure from exercise and BMR together; then, to obtain total energy expenditure, DIT will simply need to be added in).

If, for example, an athlete's BMR was calculated to be 1,750 kcal per day (7,315 kJ per day), you would multiply 1,750 kcal by 10% (0.10) to obtain DIT, which would be 175 kcal per day (732 kJ per day). Then, multiply BMR (in this case, 1,750 kcal) by one of the activity factors. In this example, we will use an activity factor of 1.550. Thus, 1,750 × 1.550 = 2,712.5 (round up to 2,713) kcal per day (11,338 kJ per day). Total energy expenditure = 2,713 (11,340 kJ) + 175 kcal (732 kJ) from DIT = 2,888 kcal per day (12,072 kJ per day).

Dietary Guidelines

In 2005 the U.S. Department of Agriculture and the U.S. Department of Health and Human Services released *Dietary Guidelines for Americans 2005*, which outlines the American government's most recent dietary and physical activity recommendations. These guidelines are similar to those of other countries. Recall that the energy equivalent of 1 lb (0.45 kg) is 3,500 kcal (14,630 kJ), meaning the body must be in a 3,500 kcal (14,630 kJ) deficit to lose 1 lb. The simplest way to create an energy deficit is to combine a decrease in energy intake with an increase in energy expenditure. For example, it is typically, but not always, easier for a person to abstain from consuming one item (for example, a candy bar) and walk for 15 minutes than it is for that person either to alter his or her diet only (by removing more than one candy bar) or to exercise only (by exercising longer than 15 minutes). The goal is to optimize the type of weight lost (primarily fat rather than fluids and lean body mass), which is the main reason for combining decreased energy intake with increased energy expenditure.

Dietary Guidelines for Americans provides some energy-lowering strategies, such as decreasing overall sugar, saturated fat, and alcohol intake while focusing on consuming low-energy foods (fruits, vegetables, soups, and so forth), whole-grain foods, and water throughout the day. Besides providing a lower amount of energy, these foods provide a much higher amount of nutrition. Fruits and vegetables in particular are nutrient-dense, low-energy foods that all people should include in their diet. People should strive to consume from five to seven servings of fruits and vegetables (combined, not five to seven servings of each) per day.

Decreasing portion sizes of meals and snacks can be an effective way to lose body weight. In many countries, particularly in the United States, portion sizes have increased by 200% or more. Because this increase has occurred gradually over the years, many people have not noticed the change. People have become accustomed to ordering a 16 oz (450 g) steak at a restaurant. Using the proper serving size of 2 to 3 oz, that single steak should be enough for six to eight people! Therefore, a gradual decrease in portion sizes is needed. People may need some time to reacquaint themselves with sensible portion sizes.

People should take time to read food labels carefully. Food labels can be misleading. For example, an item packaged in twos may have a label that provides information for only one. A person may then eat two servings while thinking that he or she has consumed one. Teaching clients to read food labels is important. After a person becomes accustomed to reading labels, doing so will take only a few seconds.

People should self-monitor their food intake as well. Although self-monitoring has its limitations, particularly for those who are overweight or obese, who tend to underreport their dietary intake (Heymsfield et al., 1995), several studies have demonstrated its effectiveness in enhancing weight loss (Boutelle & Kirschenbaum, 1998). Self-monitoring can be as simple as recording total dietary intake per day in a journal or noting the activity that may have accompanied eating. Self-

monitoring enhances accountability. This act of writing down and then seeing the list of foods and total energy consumed each day is beneficial for a person who is trying to lose weight. He or she will become more aware of the types and amounts of food consumed and will be more likely to change behavior as a result (with some nutritional counseling). See figure 6.3 for a sample food diary form that you can photocopy and give to your clients.

Macronutrient Recommendations

People are always looking for the magic bullet when it comes to weight loss. Unfortunately, these bullets are not magical, and those who try every new way of losing weight are bound to become frustrated. The low-carbohydrate fad was launched in the early 1970s, but it did not catch on then as it has in recent years. Sandwiched between the two periods of popularity of the low-carbohydrate diet was the low-fat fad that was popularized in the 1980s and then challenged in the 1990s, when the low-carbohydrate diet resurfaced. Although researchers have investigated both low-carbohydrate diets and low-fat diets, they have come to the same conclusion: An energy deficit will cause weight loss, whether it is low carbohydrate or low fat. In addition, it appears that the low-carbohydrate diet may not maintain a heart-healthy profile in the long term. Nonetheless, lower carbohydrate intakes (although not as low as diets like the Atkins diet recommend) may be helpful for some people, especially those with diabetes mellitus. Treating each person as the individual that he or she is will allow the registered dietitian to compose the proper diet plan. To be clear, we are not promoting a low-carbohydrate diet, or any diet for that matter. We are promoting a healthy diet that a person can consume for a lifetime and that helps him or her have a good metabolic profile. See chapter 7 for an in-depth discussion about low-carbohydrate diets.

In reality, creating dietary prescriptions should not be that difficult. Energy intake and energy expenditure do count; there is no way around this law of thermodynamics. Weight loss will occur if energy intake is less than energy expenditure. Ledikwe, Ello-Martin, and Rolls (2005) have shown that portions of food are increasing in conjunction with the obesity epidemic. In their review, the researchers discussed the importance of not only decreasing the consumption of high-

Daily Food Diary

Daily food or beverage amount and description	Calories	Fat
Totals		

Weekly Food Totals

	Calories	Fat
Sunday		
Monday		
Tuesday		
Wednesday		
Thursday		
Friday		
Saturday		
Totals		

Daily Exercise Diary

Daily exercise description	Duration

Weekly Exercise Totals

	Aerobic	Strength	Minutes
Sunday			
Monday			
Tuesday			
Wednesday			
Thursday			
Friday			
Saturday			
Total aerobic minutes			
Total strength minutes			

Figure 6.3 To use the daily food diary, enter the foods and amounts of each food consumed. Then enter the total kcal from the foods and the total kcal from fat. These can by obtained from nutrition labels, online, or a basic nutrition book. Enter daily totals to calculate weekly totals. For exercise, describe the type and duration of activity, then use daily totals to calculate weekly totals.

From S.L. Volpe, S.B. Sabelawski, and C.R. Mohr, 2007, *Fitness nutrition for special dietary needs* (Champaign, IL: Human Kinetics).

Sample Meal Plan for Weight Management

This sample meal plan provides a healthy variety of nutrients, food choices, vitamins, and minerals. You should work with each client individually to determine what may work for him or her, given the person's energy needs, food preferences, allergies, gender, age, and so on. No single diet can suit the needs of everyone; therefore, we provide sample meal plans as a guide within each chapter.

Breakfast

- 1 cup of oatmeal or 1 cup of whole-grain cereal = 115 g
- 1 cup of skim milk, soy milk, or rice milk = 240 ml
- 1 cup of strawberries, blueberries, or black-berries = 60 g
- 1/2 cup of orange juice or other 100% juice = 120 ml
- 1 cup of black coffee or 1 cup hot tea = 240 ml

Snack

- 1 medium orange, peach, or apple = 80 g
- 2 oz of unsalted mixed nuts = 56 g
- 12 oz of water = 360 ml

Lunch

- Turkey sandwich
  - 2 oz of sliced turkey breast (not processed) = 56 g
  - 2 slices of whole-wheat bread = 80 g
  - 2 slices each of lettuce and tomato = 45 g
  - 1 tsp of mustard = 5 g
- 1 cup of mixed greens salad = 220 g
- 1 tbsp of vinaigrette dressing = 15 g
- 1 cup of skim milk = 240 ml

Snack

- 1/2 cup of fat-free cottage cheese = 120 g
- 12 oz of water = 360 ml

Dinner

- 3 oz of baked salmon = 90 g
- 1/2 cup of brown rice = 115 g
- 1/2 cup of steamed asparagus = 115 g
- 1 whole-wheat dinner roll = 80 g
- 1 cup of skim milk = 240 ml

Snack

- 6 oz of vanilla low-fat yogurt = 140 g
- 1 medium peach = 80 g
- 12 oz of water = 360 ml

This sample meal plan provides at least 100% of the Dietary Reference Intakes (DRIs) for energy, protein, fiber, vitamins A, C, E, B_6, B_{12}, thiamin, riboflavin, niacin, folate, calcium, iron, magnesium, phosphorus, zinc (Food and Nutrition Board (1997, 1998, 2005), and approximately

- 2,000 kcal (8,360 kJ),
- 103 g of protein,
- 93 g of fat,
- 31 g of fiber, and
- 2,500 mg of sodium.

From S.L. Volpe, S.B. Sabelawski, and C.R. Mohr, 2007, *Fitness nutrition for special dietary needs* (Champaign, IL: Human Kinetics).

energy, high-fat foods but also increasing the consumption of low-energy, low-fat foods, such as fruits and vegetables. Ledikwe and colleagues noted that focusing on the positive message of increasing the consumption of healthful foods might be more important than focusing on eliminating or reducing the intake of less healthful, high-energy foods.

People should follow a diet within the Acceptable Macronutrient Distribution Ranges (AMDR) for fat, carbohydrate, and protein established under the Dietary Reference Intakes (DRIs) (Food and Nutrition Board, 2005). The following are the AMDRs for adults for each of the macronutrients.

- Carbohydrate: 5% to 65% of total energy intake
- Protein: 10% to 35% of total energy intake
- Fat: 20% to 35% of total energy intake

These percentages should be altered to meet individual needs. For example, people who are active may need to consume a greater amount of carbohydrate than their sedentary counterparts do. Focusing on or eliminating a food group or several food groups limits a person's ability to obtain all the necessary nutrients. Therefore, restrictive diets are not recommended for long-term use. Diets should focus on both quantity and quality. Research has even suggested that adding fruits and vegetables rather than focusing on eliminating foods enhances weight loss. The sample meal plan for weight management provides a guideline for people who are active and trying to lose weight.

DIETARY SUPPLEMENTS AND WEIGHT LOSS

Obesity is a complex disease that encompasses a number of physiological and psychological aspects. Successful weight loss entails not only dietary and activity modifications, as discussed, but also behavioral changes. As a last resort and for the morbidly obese, pharmacological or surgical treatments are sometimes required. Many people turn to dietary supplements with the hope of enhancing weight-loss efforts. Most supplements do not help with weight loss. The following section, based on published research, discusses purported weight-loss supplements and their effects, if any.

The Federal Trade Commission (2002) reported that in the year 2000, U.S. consumers spent approximately US$35 billion on weight-loss products (books, dietary supplements, weight-loss franchises, and so on). People want instant results; dietary supplements are attractive because advertisements promise to deliver what they are seeking.

Caffeine

Caffeine is the cornerstone of many fat-loss supplements because of its well-documented effects on thermogenesis and *lipolysis* (Acheson et al., 2004; Acheson, Zahorska-Markiewicz, Pittet, Anantharaman, & Jequier, 1980; Arciero, Gardner, Calles-Escandon, Benowitz, & Poehlman, 1995; Astrup, Toubro, Christensen, & Quaade, 1992; Bracco, Ferrarra, Arnaud, Jequier, & Schutz, 1995). Caffeine, however, is rarely used as a stand-alone product to enhance fat loss. Instead, it is typically a component of a proprietary formula that makes up the product.

Caffeine stimulates energy expenditure through increased sympathetic nervous system stimulation (Bellet, Roman, DeCastro, Kim, & Kershbaum, 1969). Results from in vitro studies demonstrate that caffeine may also work synergistically with adrenaline to enhance lipolysis (Butcher, Baird, & Sutherland, 1968). Therefore, it seems to exert its effects in a variety of ways, not solely through stimulation of the sympathetic nervous system.

High doses of caffeine can have some negative side effects. Caffeine may elevate blood pressure and heart rate (Debrah, Haigh, Sherwin, Murphy, & Kerr, 1995). One study reported that high doses of caffeine may elicit loose bowels or diarrhea. A regular cup of coffee contains approximately 100 mg of caffeine (which will vary with bean type, length of brewing, and so on; in comparison, one cup of tea contains about 50 mg of caffeine). For regular consumers of caffeine, intakes greater than usual are not recommended. Those who are caffeine naive can experience anxiety, increased heart rate, and other effects if they consume caffeine above their usual zero to small intake. Such people should be cautious about taking even moderate doses of caffeine. Some weight-loss products provide several hundred milligrams of caffeine, which is above what a person may normally consume throughout the day.

As a side note, scientists have argued over the years about the risks and benefits of coffee drinking (not caffeine per say). Pereira, Parker, and Folsom (2006) reported that decaffeinated coffee intake of 6 or more cups per day resulted in a 22% reduction in the relative risk of type 2 diabetes mellitus in women who were studied over an 11-year period. We share the results of this recent study not because we recommend that people start to consume large quantities of decaffeinated coffee, but because we want health care professionals to keep their clients' likes and dislikes in mind during nutrition counseling, and keep abreast of recent research in physical activity and nutrition.

Carnitine

Carnitine has been popular as a weight-loss supplement because of its mechanism of action; carnitine is necessary to shuttle fatty acids into the mitochondria for oxidation. Therefore, in theory, carnitine would be useful as an adjunct to a healthy diet and exercise regimen to enhance weight loss. Villani, Gannon, Self, and Rich (2000) reported that carnitine was not effective in enhancing weight loss. This particular study included 36 premenopausal women who received either 2 g of L-carnitine per day or a placebo. Throughout the 8-week study, all participants were assigned to perform moderate aerobic exercise for 30 minutes per day, 4 days per week. At the end of the study, no differences were found between groups in body weight, fat mass, or resting lipid utilization. Moreover, five of the subjects in the L-carnitine group dropped out of the study because of nausea or diarrhea. A review paper published the same year drew the same conclusion and suggested that little or no evidence supports the use of carnitine for weight loss in humans (Dyck, 2000).

Chitosan

Chitosan is believed to decrease the amount of fat absorbed and digested (Mhurchu et al., 2004). Chitosan advertisements have even stated that dietary changes are unnecessary when supplementing with chitosan. It is purported to work by binding and trapping dietary fat, causing fat to be excreted, resulting in weight loss. Although this sounds promising in theory, the results of the studies published on chitosan are equivocal. In addition, people who are allergic to shellfish may have a similar allergic reaction to chitosan, because it is extracted from the shells of shellfish (Guerciolini, Radu-Radulescu, Boldrin, Dallas, & Moore, 2001).

A recent study published by Gades and Stern (2005) suggested that treatment with chitosan did not result in significant excretion of fat compared with taking a placebo. This short, 12-day study with 24 male and female subjects found that when subjects consumed 2.5 grams per day of chitosan with a meal, they experienced no significant change in the amount of fat "trapped and excreted." This short-duration study was not designed to determine whether subjects lost weight, but rather to assess whether chitosan did in fact trap and excrete fat, as claimed by advertisements. Indeed, it did not. Other researchers have also reported that chitosan does not trap and excrete fat and does not result in significant weight loss (Mhurchu, Dunshea-Mooij, Bennett, & Rodgers, 2005a, 2005b).

Chromium

Chromium is an essential trace mineral widely used in fat-loss supplements. According to a report in 1999, approximately 10 million Americans took chromium supplements and spent about US$150 million per year on the ingredient, making chromium the second-largest-selling mineral after calcium (Hellerstein, 1998). This occurred despite the fact that many well-conducted studies about chromium have not supported its claims as a weight-loss agent.

Volpe, Huang, Larpadisorn, and Lesser (2001) assessed the effects of supplementation with 400 μg per day of chromium picolinate compared with a placebo on body composition, resting metabolic rate, strength, and several other biochemical parameters. The subjects in this study were 44 moderately obese women who were assigned, in a double-blind manner, to receive chromium or an identical-looking placebo. Both groups participated in supervised resistance-training and walking regimens, 2 days per week for 12 weeks. At the end of the 12 weeks, supplementation with 400 μg per day of chromium picolinate had no significant effects on any of the outcome parameters measured: body composition, resting metabolic rate, or strength (Volpe et al., 2001). A more recent review of several dietary supplements drew the same conclusion: Chromium supplementation cannot be recommended for weight loss (Pittler & Ernst, 2004). Note, however, that some evidence indicates that chromium supplementation may be effective as a treatment for type 2 diabetes mellitus. Studies are ongoing, so additional publications on this topic should be forthcoming.

Citrus Aurantium

With the banning of ephedra in weight loss products, sales of Citrus aurantium (or synephrine, the most active ingredient in Citrus aurantium) have skyrocketed. Citrus aurantium, also known

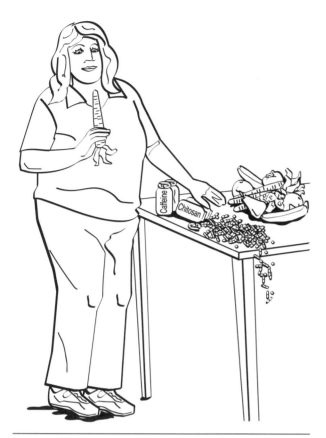

Figure 6.4 Although many people would prefer to use pills to "melt away" fat, these methods usually do not work. The best way to lose weight and maintain healthy body weight is to eat healthy foods and exercise.

as bitter, or seville, orange, is a small citrus tree. Its most active components are synephrine and octopamine, but synephrine is typically in higher concentration than octopamine is. Synephrine stimulates the β-adrenergic receptors. Briefly, β-receptors are located throughout the body, and four separate subtypes have been classified: β-1, β-2, β-3, and β-4 (Mutlu, Koch, & Factor, 2004) The β-3 receptors are found mostly in fat cells and are thought to be responsible for the thermogenic effects within the body. The β-1 and β-2 receptors are located mostly in the alveolar walls of the lungs. The β-4 receptors seem to be a type of β-1 receptor, except they are located primarily in the myocardial cells (Mutlu et al.).

Haaz et al. (2006) reviewed the available literature on synephrine for safety and efficacy. These scientists offered the judgment that although some results are promising, larger, more well-controlled trials need to be conducted before any

conclusions can be drawn about the safety and efficacy of synephrine. Other reviews have come to similar conclusions; more well-controlled studies in this area are needed before this herb can be recommended for weight loss (Bent, Padula, & Neuhaus, 2004). Studies conducted in humans either lacked adequate controls or did not use synephrine as an independent determinant for weight loss. Therefore, definitive conclusions cannot be made.

Coleus Forskohlii

Coleus forskohlii is an herb that has been used since ancient times to treat heart and respiratory disorders. More recently, it has been added to weight-loss products. Herbal product manufacturers are now producing Coleus forskohlii extracts with elevated levels of the constituent forskolin.

One recent published study, however, evaluated the effects of 50 g of Coleus forskohlii extract per kg of body weight in ovariectomized rats (Han, Morimoto, Yu, & Okuda, 2005). The researchers reported that the rats supplemented with Coleus forskohlii had reduced body weight, food intake, and fat accumulation. Extrapolating these findings to humans is impossible, however, and research on forskolin in humans is limited.

One pilot study provided six overweight women with 250 mg of Coleus forskohlii, standardized to provide 10% (25 mg) of forskolin twice daily for 12 weeks (Kreider et al., 2002). The authors found no statistical difference between those supplementing with Coleus forskohlii and those supplementing with the placebo in body weight or body fat over the 12-week period. Another study published in *Obesity Research* in 2005 examined the effect of forskolin on various parameters, including body composition and resting metabolic rate (RMR), in overweight and obese (BMI ≥ 26 kg/m^2) men. In this double blind, placebo-controlled trial, 15 men were given 250 mg of forskolin, and 15 men were given placebo twice per day, for 12 weeks. Those in the forskolin group had statistically significant decreases in fat mass (kg) when compared to the placebo group, but there were no differences in RMR between groups. The authors suggested that long-term reserch is warranted to truly ascertain the effects of this herb. Moreover, its safety and efficacy are concerns; Baumann,

Felix, Sattelberger, and Klein (1990) reported that it may worsen cardiovascular conditions by causing vasodilation and lowering blood pressure. Although we do not want to sound like a broken record, additional randomized, double-blind, placebo-controlled studies on this herb are required before definitive statements can be made on its safety and efficacy as a weight-loss supplement.

Conjugated Linoleic Acid

Conjugated linoleic acid (CLA) has been proposed as a way to increase metabolic rate and fat utilization, and thus, to enhance weight loss (Pariza & Ha, 1990). Linoleic acid is an essential fatty acid, meaning that the body requires exogenous intake of this fat. CLA is found primarily in dairy products (not in skimmed dairy products) and meat, specifically, beef and lamb (Ritzenthaler et al., 2001). The typical dietary intake is approximately 212 mg per day for men and 151 mg per day for women (Ritzenthaler et al.; Terpstra, 2004).

CLA has been studied for various effects on health, including its effects on body composition and weight loss. Like many fat-loss supplements, CLA has produced positive results in studies of body composition of animals. These positive results, however, have not been consistently reported in humans; most researchers have reported no change in body composition with CLA supplementation in humans. Furthermore, CLA may have negative effects on blood lipid levels and glucose levels (Riserus, Smedman, Basu, & Vessby, 2003), although these results have been equivocal.

In a meta-analysis published in the *American Journal of Clinical Nutrition*, Terpstra (2004) reviewed the few human studies conducted on CLA published as full-length articles in peer-reviewed journals. Discrepancy has appeared in the literature regarding dosing; some studies have used as little as 1.4 g of CLA per day (approximately 6 times the normal dietary intake for men), and others have used up to 6.8 g of CLA per day (approximately 30 times the normal dietary intake for men). In this meta-analysis, none of the studies reviewed found a significant reduction in body weight; only two studies showed a significant, but small, decrease in body fat.

The data in animals do appear promising, but the doses used in the animal studies are not applicable to humans. For example, when evaluating CLA supplementation as a percentage of total energy, animal studies that have demonstrated a positive effect from CLA supplementation have provided approximately 0.70 g of CLA per kg of body weight, whereas human studies (such as those described earlier) provided approximately 0.04 g of CLA per kg of body weight (Malpuech-Brugere et al., 2004). For humans, the same relative dose of CLA used in the animal studies would be over 50 g of CLA per day (varying accordingly with body weight). This dosage level is not cost-effective and may be harmful because CLA has been shown to be a pro-oxidant. Further, recent research has suggested that CLA may cause insulin resistance in obese men (Riserus, Vessby, Arnlov, & Basu, 2004). More research is warranted to clarify these findings.

Green Tea

Green tea, which has recently gained popularity in the United States, is the most widely consumed beverage in the world, second only to water (Chantre & Lairon, 2002). Much research has evaluated green tea as a beverage for weight loss and general health. Green tea, by increasing metabolic rate, has shown promise as an adjunct to an effective diet and exercise regimen in some studies (Dulloo et al., 1999), but not all studies are in agreement with its potential effects on weight loss (Diepvens, Kovacs, Nijs, Vogels, & Westerterp-Plantenga, 2005).

Green tea is a good source of catechins. Green tea contains four catechins, but the one that has been shown to be beneficial for weight loss is called epigallocatechin-3-gallate (EGCG). With respect to weight loss, EGCG and the naturally occurring caffeine in green tea appear to have a synergistic relationship; the two together may increase thermogenesis (Dulloo et al., 1999). Brewed green tea provides approximately 10 to 80 mg of caffeine and 50 to 100 mg of EGCG per cup, but these numbers can increase when using extracts of the product.

Dulloo et al. (1999) conducted a pilot study to determine whether green tea extract had any effect on resting metabolic rate. The researchers provided subjects with one of three supplements: (1) green tea extract (providing 270 mg of EGCG and 150 mg of caffeine per day), (2) 150 mg of caffeine per day, or (3) a placebo to determine whether the thermogenic effect resulted from EGCG itself or from combining with caffeine. The results of this 24-hour study suggested that the EGCG plus caffeine significantly increased resting metabolic rate by 4%. This result could not be correlated with any body-weight changes because of the short duration of the study.

Diepvens et al. (2005) assessed the effects of green tea, which provided 1,125 mg of tea catechins and 225 mg of caffeine per day, versus a placebo. All subjects were fed a low-energy diet throughout the study, so the variable was the addition of the green tea. Results of the study demonstrated a reduction in body weight in both groups, with no significant differences between the green tea and the placebo. Body mass index, waist-to-hip ratio, fat mass, and fat-free mass were not significantly different between groups. The researchers concluded that the green tea provided no additive benefit to a low-energy diet on body weight or body composition.

Some research has suggested that tea as a beverage, as opposed to just the extract, may be of benefit. Thus, another component of the beverage may be beneficial, a topic that should be explored (Wu et al., 2003). Disregarding the body-weight issue, regular consumption of green tea has been shown to provide numerous other health benefits if known contraindications, such as use of coumadin, are not present (Booth, Madabushi, Davidson, & Sadowski, 1995; Taylor & Wilt, 1999). Some literature suggests that green tea may mimic the actions of antiplatelet prescription medications, such as coumadin, so harm could occur if the two are consumed together (Son et al., 2004).

Double-blind, placebo-controlled, randomized longitudinal studies are necessary to determine the effects, if any, of green tea on body weight and body composition. In addition, research needs to be conducted to evaluate whether consumption of green tea promotes weight loss better than consumption of green tea extract does.

Hydroxycitric Acid (HCA)

HCA is produced from the rind of the fruit of Garcinia cambogia, which is native to India and popular as a food additive in Asian cultures (van Loon et al., 2000). HCA is now commonly included in weight-loss aids, particularly because research in animals has suggested that it promotes weight loss, in part through suppression of hunger. But few well-controlled studies on humans have assessed the claims; most of the supportive literature has been conducted in rodents.

Mattes and Bormann (2000) published a study measuring the effects of HCA on appetite and hunger in overweight adults. In this 12-week, double-blind, randomized controlled trial, the authors attempted to ascertain the mechanism behind the use of HCA for weight loss and, more specifically, appetite control. Forty-two of the 89 subjects in this study ingested 400 mg caplets of Garcinia cambogia, 30 to 60 minutes before meals, providing 1.2 g of HCA per day, and 47 subjects received a placebo. All participants were prescribed a 1,200 kcal diet. Mattes and Bormann reported significant weight loss over the 12-week period, but the differences between the HCA and placebo groups were not statistically significant. Furthermore, the HCA group did not exhibit better dietary adherence or appetite suppression compared with the control group. Thus, it does not appear that HCA is an effective supplement for weight loss.

A more recent review of a number of dietary supplements purported to enhance weight loss was published in the *American Journal of Clinical Nutrition* (Pittler & Ernst, 2004). HCA was among the supplements considered in this review. The conclusion by the authors was that none of the dietary supplements reviewed for weight loss could be recommended because the data were not convincing regarding the effect of any over-the-counter weight-loss product. Table 6.5 provides a summary of the supplements discussed in this chapter.

The incidence of obesity continues to increase rapidly worldwide. Subsequently, dietary supplements intended to enhance weight loss will continue to be popular, despite the lack of positive results from peer-reviewed research. Even if supplements produce a small positive effect, a balanced diet with a modest energy reduction and an increase in energy expenditure can more safely achieve the same result. Consulting with a physician before taking any dietary supplement is always recommended, especially if a person is taking prescribed medications or has any chronic illness or allergies. Overall, the risk–benefit ratio of taking supplements to lose weight is high—that

Table 6.5   Fat-Loss Supplements and Their Purported Mechanisms

Ingredient	Purported mechanism	Scientific evidence
Caffeine	Enhances lipolysis and thermogenesis by inhibiting enzymes that may otherwise stop the process.	Caffeine has moderate effects on lipolysis. Caffeine alone, however, will not cause a decrease in body weight.
Carnitine	Necessary to shuttle fatty acids into the mitochondria for oxidation.	Although carnitine is necessary for fatty acid oxidation, supplementing with excess carnitine does not appear to enhance this process further.
Chitosan	Binds to negatively charged fat in the intestine for excretion.	Supportive animal data have not shown carryover to efficacy in humans.
Chromium	Stimulates insulin, which will enhance glucose and fat metabolism in the body. Will also enhance lean body mass.	Although chromium does appear to enhance insulin sensitivity, it has not shown promise in weight-loss studies.
Citrus aurantium	Enhances fat loss by acting primarily on β-3 receptors, which are responsible for lipolytic and thermogenic effects.	No studies have measured the independent effects of Citrus aurantium on weight loss.
Coleus forskohlii	This herb may possibly suppress appetite and enhance the utilization of fatty acids in the body.	Without any peer-reviewed studies to date on this single ingredient for weight loss, assessing the validity of the claims is impossible.
Conjugated linoleic acid (CLA)	Increases metabolic rate and fat utilization.	Research in humans has not supported the claims.
Green tea (epigallocatechin-3-gallate, or EGCG)	One of the catechins in green tea, EGCG may prolong thermogenesis and increase fat metabolism. It may also aid in fat utilization and metabolism.	Some evidence has demonstrated that EGCG may enhance thermogenesis; longer-term studies need to be conducted to ascertain the efficacy.
Hydroxycitric acid	Inhibits an enzyme that would otherwise slow lipogenesis, which would help the body burn fat longer.	Data in animals are promising, but the data in humans are not supportive.

From S.L. Volpe, S.B. Sabelawski, and C.R. Mohr, 2007, *Fitness nutrition for special dietary needs* (Champaign, IL: Human Kinetics).

is, it is not worth the money or risk to take supplements for weight loss that have not been shown to be effective. A person would do better by saving his or her money to buy healthier foods, join a gym or exercise classes, or buy a good pair of walking shoes.

PHYSICAL ACTIVITY

Although many interactions occur between the environment and genetics, and although morbidly obese people need surgery or pharmaceutical treatments, weight loss for most people is ultimately a result of decreasing energy intake and increasing energy expenditure. Tipping the energy balance in the negative direction may not produce quick results, but done properly it will lead to a safe, healthy weight loss over time that minimizes loss of lean body mass. Combining daily physical activity with a healthy diet that provides the required nutrients and can be consumed for a lifetime is vital for weight-loss success and long-term maintenance of a healthy weight.

Aerobic Exercise

Depending on their level of overweight and obesity, some people have a difficult time increasing their energy expenditure through regular physical activity because of their excess weight and poor fitness. Studies have demonstrated, however, that people are more likely to adopt exercise long term if they begin to exercise at the onset of their weight-loss effort. Walking is one of the simplest forms of exercise, but any form of moderate-intensity exercise will suffice. Knowing that most people who are overweight or obese are also sedentary, clinicians should initially encourage overweight and obese adults to perform at least 150 minutes of moderately intense exercise each week (30 minutes per day on 5 days of the week), because this level of exercise has been shown to improve health-related outcomes (Jakicic, 2003b). This amount of exercise, however, may not be enough to enhance weight loss and facilitate weight maintenance. Studies have demonstrated that higher levels of exercise may be necessary to enhance long-term weight loss and maintenance (Jakicic, 2003a, 2003b). Not surprisingly, those who exercised the most minutes per week lost more weight than those who exercised less (Jakicic, 2003a, 2003b).

The most recent statement from the Institute of Medicine recommends that people progressively increase exercise of moderate to vigorous intensity to approximately 60 minutes per day on most days of the week to help manage body weight and prevent weight gain. To sustain weight loss in adulthood, the recommendation is to participate in 60 to 90 minutes of moderate-intensity to vigorous physical activity most days of the week. Although sedentary people may view this as an unreachable goal, you should counsel clients that engaging in 60 to 90 minutes of physical activity each day is a long-term goal that they should not expect to attain at the initiation of an exercise program. Consider suggesting a stepwise program in which they begin exercising for 15 minutes on 5 days of the week for 4 weeks, then do 20 minutes on 5 days of the week for 4 weeks, and so on until they reach the ultimate goal. Remind clients that they need not perform their daily exercise in a single session; research has shown that 10-minute bouts accumulated throughout the day are just as effective for weight loss and improving fitness as extended bouts (Jakicic, Wing, Butler, & Robertson, 1995). People who have a varied schedule may find a multiple-bout exercise approach easier to fit into their daily set of activities, thus

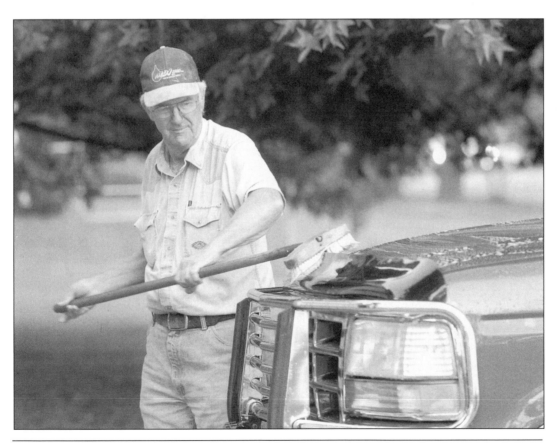

Sedentary adults should be encouraged to consider active daily living tasks as part of their exercise program. Everything from washing trucks and mowing lawns to parking a little farther back in the store parking lot than usual can be counted.

increasing the likelihood that they will adhere to an exercise program. Encourage the use of devices such as pedometers to facilitate exercise adoption (Jakicic, 2003b). Furthermore, promote lifestyle activities (such as taking the stairs, taking a parking space farther from the door, and mowing the lawn with a push mower) that will expend energy throughout the day.

Resistance Training

Besides increasing energy expenditure during a weight-loss program, exercise is intended to reduce the normal decrease in lean body mass that occurs during a reduction in energy intake. This decrease cannot be prevented with aerobic exercise activity alone, especially because the level of lean body mass previously necessary to carry an overweight or obese person is no longer necessary with the decrease in overall body mass. Nonetheless, preserving lean body mass is as important as losing weight. The goal with any weight-loss regimen is to improve overall body composition (less fat, more lean body mass) rather than to focus solely on total body-weight loss.

The primary role of resistance training is to increase or maintain lean body mass. In addition, resistance training protects joints, which can decrease the risk of injury. Both functions are important, especially for a person who may have been sedentary for his or her entire life and who may be prone to injury.

More information on resistance training as a component of a weight-loss program will be provided in the exercise prescription section.

To date, most research that has examined various exercise modalities and weight loss has not demonstrated that resistance exercise provides a significant benefit over aerobic exercise. Theoretically, resistance exercise may be beneficial through its effect on resting metabolic rate (RMR) and fat-free mass, but the research in this area thus far has been equivocal. The recent position stand of the American College of Sports Medicine on appropriate intervention strategies for weight loss and prevention of weight regain for adults (Jakicic et al., 2001) suggests that resistance training is not the most effective means for weight loss. Resistance training may indeed increase RMR, but this potential increase in RMR has not been shown to offset the reductions in RMR typically experienced through weight-loss intervention programs (Geliebter et al., 1997; Wadden et al., 1997).

Donnelly et al. (1993) examined the role of resistance exercise in a weight-loss program using very low energy diets (VLEDs). The results from this study demonstrated that subjects in the weight-training group demonstrated muscle fiber hypertrophy and strength gains compared with the nonexercising group, when following a VLED. But weight training did not affect the total amount of weight or fat-free mass lost in the exercising group compared with the nonexercising group. Thus, despite an increase in

---

Myths for Weight Management: Spot Reduction

A common belief is that a person can perform sit-ups daily to decrease the size of his or her abdomen. This activity is known as spot reduction, but it does not work. A person cannot exercise one part of the body and expect fat loss to occur in that particular area. If a person wants to strengthen his or her abdominal muscles, or any other muscles, resistance training can accomplish it. But working a particular area of the body anaerobically will not reduce fat in that area. So how can a person reduce fat in a certain area? Exercising aerobically (walking, swimming, running, cross-country skiing, and so on) will burn fat throughout the body. By utilizing fat throughout the body, fat will be lost in the particular area of interest. Nonetheless, genetics will have an influence on the amount of fat lost in a particular area. For example, if a person's family members all deposit most of their fat in their hips or gluteal region, that person will be able to lose fat from that area but at a slower rate than a person whose family does not deposit fat in the hips or gluteal region. A sound aerobic exercise program combined with weight training to strengthen and maintain muscle mass is what will help attain weight loss and maintain a healthy weight.

Sample Exercise Prescription for Weight Management

- Depending on the baseline level of fitness and body weight, people should gradually progress to higher levels of exercise over time.

- Behavioral strategies can be effective in helping people adopt higher levels of exercise. Devices such as pedometers are helpful in motivating people to exercise.

- Aerobic exercise should be increased in a stepwise manner, every 4 weeks, until the person reaches his or her goal of 60 to 90 minutes per day on most, preferably all, days of the week. Depending on the individual, more time or different goals may be appropriate.

- Resistance training is an important adjunct to a sound program based on aerobic exercise. Basic instruction in resistance training is important. The trainer should stress the importance of breathing, using proper form during weightlifting to train the intended

muscle, and using a weight that the person can move comfortably for 10 to 12 repetitions. Ultimately, the person will be able to increase the resistance, number of sets performed, and variety of exercises. Weight-training machines are usually safer to use than free weights, but free weights provide greater range of motion. Either way, a person who is qualified in the area of resistance training should assist the person for the first several sessions.

- For some people, the most important function of resistance training may be strengthening large-muscle groups. If a person is unable to get out of a chair, recommending aerobic exercise is nonsensical. This person must first work to increase overall strength.

- To increase activities of daily living, people can park farther from the store, take the stairs instead of the elevator, and so on.

strength and muscle fiber size, weight training was unable to preserve the loss of fat-free mass often seen during weight loss. Remember, however, that if a 300 lb (136 kg) person loses 50 total lb (23 kg), for example, he or she does not need as much fat-free body mass to bear the weight of his or her body because overall body mass has decreased significantly.

In another study, Bryner et al. (1999) compared resistance training with aerobic training on lean body mass and RMR when subjects were consuming a VLED. They reported a positive increase in RMR and maintenance of fat-free mass in the resistance-trained group over the 12-week period. But they reported no significant difference in fat-free mass between groups at the end of the 12 weeks, despite greater total weight loss in the group that did aerobic training versus the group that did resistance training (19.4% versus 14.7% decrease in body weight, respectively).

Data from research protocols using VLEDs should not be generalized to more common situations in which people moderately decrease energy intake and increase energy output. The results do demonstrate, however, that under extreme energy restriction, subjects are unable to

prevent the loss of fat-free mass that commonly occurs during weight loss. In addition, many overweight sedentary people are unwilling to begin and sustain a structured resistance exercise program because it may be unfamiliar to them. Therefore, participation in home-based aerobic exercise programs (for example, walking) may be more appropriate and has shown to be effective in promoting adoption and maintenance of regular exercise (King, Haskell, Taylor, Kraemer, & DeBusk, 1991; Perri, Martin, Leermakers, Sears, & Notelovitz, 1997), thus potentially having greater long-term effect on overall weight loss.

Although both aerobic and anaerobic training play a role in an overall healthful lifestyle, resistance training by itself should not be recommended as a means for weight loss because the research has clearly demonstrated otherwise. Those engaging in weight-loss efforts should be encouraged to begin an exercise regimen within their abilities, while being aware of their limitations. An exercise program will ultimately enhance a person's ability to perform activities of daily living because he or she will be able to move more freely and comfortably with the decrease in overall body mass.

CASE STUDY

Our guest dietitian in this chapter is one of the authors, who has experience working with behavioral weight-loss interventions. This client needed to lose weight because he was having difficulties with simple activities of daily living.

C.R. was a 245 lb (111 kg) 35-year-old man. He had a BMI of 34, which put him in the moderately obese category (class I), on the borderline of becoming severely obese (class II). He was interested in weight loss because he recently noticed that his joints were aching, he was having difficulty performing everyday tasks because he was too fatigued, and he could no longer walk up the two flights of stairs at work without stopping after the first flight to catch his breath. He was not aware that he had any other physiological abnormalities, and his recent blood work indicated that everything was within normal limits. Nonetheless, he had a strong family history of cardiovascular disease: His father and both uncles died of myocardial infarctions (heart attacks) before age 45.

In a meeting, C.R. and I discussed a typical day for him at the office and at home. Was he active? How could he make time for activity? Did he have a supportive family? We also discussed his general eating patterns and determined where he could make changes. As an executive at a major corporation, C.R. had a demanding schedule. He made it clear that carving out time each day for exercise would be nearly impossible.

I gave C.R. a food diary and instructed him on how to complete it properly. He agreed that he would not have a problem doing this because he could keep the diary with him at all times. Because self-monitoring has been shown to be an effective weight-management tool independent of any other change, it was important for C.R. to use the food diary on a daily basis. In addition, I gave C.R. a sample menu with examples of meals and snack foods that would provide him with 2,000 kcal (8,360 kJ) each day with less than 30% of the total energy derived from fat. These menus were in general agreement with the guidelines established by the National Institutes of Health and have been shown to be effective in such models as the National Weight Control Registry.

Although C.R. needed to decrease his energy intake by the recommended amount to achieve weight loss, it was difficult for him to put forth the effort to make the change. Therefore, we worked together to set small, attainable goals that would ultimately allow him to reach his larger goals that we discussed when he first came for assistance. We started the discussion of goals early in our counseling sessions so that C.R. would have something to work toward. He and I did not become overzealous by putting unrealistic expectations on him, such as rapid weight loss. We discussed some small goals like adding one fruit or vegetable to each day of the week. When he accomplished and was able to maintain this new eating habit, we went to two, three, and finally five servings each day. We did the same thing with decreasing soda consumption. Rather than telling C.R. to eliminate all soda from his diet, I initially asked him to cut whatever he consumed in half. Over time, as his soda dependency subsided, he could then switch to healthier beverages, such as plain water, tea, or non-fat or low-fat milk. I also continually reminded him that weight loss of as little as 5% can have a significant positive effect on health outcomes.

In addition, because C.R. was currently inactive, I gave him an exercise prescription of 20 minutes of exercise per day, 5 days per week to start. Keeping in mind his demanding schedule, we discussed the research showing that short bouts of activity are equally effective for weight loss and cardiovascular benefits, providing they accumulate to the required amount of activity. C.R. agreed that he could perform 10 minutes of physical activity before work and take 10 minutes during the day for physical activity.

Every 4 weeks he would increase the duration of his exercise by 10 minutes each day, so that in the 9th week he would be exercising 40 minutes per day, 5 days per week. The ultimate goal was to increase his total physical activity to 60 minutes per day. He stated that it would be impossible for him to carve out 40 to 60 minutes per day for steady physical activity; I therefore reiterated that short, multiple bouts of physical activity are equally effective. This approach may work best for him.

C.R. was an adherent client. Because of his work schedule and family demands, he did not want to put much time into food preparation. Thus he often used portion-controlled meals (such as frozen meals, yogurt, yogurt shakes, and fruit). He began to enjoy the way that exercise made him feel and noticed a big difference in his overall mood and demeanor afterward. Because of this positive reinforcement, he added

10 minutes of physical activity after work and subsequently added 10 more minutes when he could fit it in to his schedule, for a total of 30 to 40 minutes of physical activity, 5 days per week.

C.R. lost weight rather quickly in the beginning, about 3 to 4 lb (1.4 to 1.6 kg) per week, as is common when people start weight-loss programs. His progress began to slow later to the recommended 1 to 2 lb (0.45 to 0.9 kg) per week. By the end of 12 weeks, he had decreased his body weight by approximately 25 lb (11.4 kg). He had more energy, more focus, and greater vitality. Although he still had more weight to lose at the 12-week point to shift into the normal-weight category according to his BMI, research has shown that the 10% of initial weight that he had already lost would significantly decrease his disease risk.

After the 12-week program ended, C.R. continued to lose weight and was not satisfied until he decreased his BMI to meet the criteria for normal weight. He is now an avid exerciser, which has helped him maintain his body weight. He enjoys cycling, hiking, and running, activities that he could not dream of doing when he started the program. More important, he is performing some of his physical activity with his family, thus increasing time spent with them, while achieving his exercise goals each week.

Christopher R. Mohr, PhD, RD
President, Mohr Results, Inc.
Louisville, Kentucky

Diabetes Mellitus

The two major types of diabetes mellitus are type 1, formerly known as juvenile onset diabetes or insulin-dependent diabetes mellitus, and type 2, formerly known as adult onset or noninsulin-dependent diabetes mellitus. Type 1 diabetes mellitus occurs in about 5% to 10% of the population, whereas type 2 diabetes mellitus occurs in 90% to 95% of those who contract diabetes. Type 1 diabetes mellitus is an autoimmune disease that affects the beta cells of the pancreas, the cells that release insulin. Type 2 diabetes mellitus results from the inability of the insulin receptors to recognize insulin produced by the body. This circumstance usually occurs in people who have become obese. This chapter focuses on these two types of diabetes and on the nutritional needs of those with diabetes mellitus who exercise.

OVERVIEW OF DIABETES MELLITUS

According to the American Diabetes Association (2003), "Diabetes mellitus is a group of metabolic diseases characterized by hyperglycemia resulting from defects in insulin secretion, insulin action, or both."

In 2000 the World Health Organization (WHO) estimated worldwide occurrence of type 1 and type 2 diabetes mellitus at 171 million; WHO has

predicted that this number will increase to 366 million by 2030. In the year 2000 large numbers of people who had diabetes mellitus lived in all regions of the world:

- Africa: 7,020,000
- Eastern Mediterranean region: 15,188,000
- Europe: 33,332,000
- North and South America: 33,016,000
- Southeast Asia: 46,903,000
- Western Pacific region: 35,771,000

Refer to the World Health Organization (WHO) Web site (www.who.int/diabetes/facts/world_figures/en/index.html) to obtain prevalence for specific countries within each of the regions.

The subsections that follow discuss the main metabolic diseases and present statistics on the worldwide prevalence of diabetes.

Type 1 Diabetes Mellitus

Type 1 diabetes mellitus typically occurs in adolescents who are genetically predisposed to this disease (Trucco, 2006). In type 1 diabetes mellitus, the beta cells of the pancreas do not produce insulin or they produce it in such small quantities that the body cannot use glucose for energy. Glucose, also called blood sugar, is produced from the breakdown of carbohydrate foods. The cause of this type of diabetes is probably an autoimmune response in which the body attacks its own pancreas, inhibiting its functionality. A virus that affects the pancreas may also cause type 1 diabetes mellitus.

Because a person with type 1 diabetes mellitus cannot produce insulin, insulin injections are required. The different forms of insulin are short acting, medium acting, and long acting. Sometimes the different forms are mixed, depending on the person and his or her control. Insulin pumps can also be useful in controlling type 1 diabetes mellitus. The pumps are worn on the hip, like a beeper or cell phone, and attach to a long catheter that can release insulin directly into the body through a small needle that is left in the skin. For people who have type 1 diabetes mellitus, using a pump is more convenient than taking multiple shots daily. Recently, some success has occurred with stem cell transplants of the pancreas, which could result in a cure for type 1 diabetes mellitus. Pancreatic islet transplantation is another viable option for some patients with type 1 diabetes mellitus, and it has resulted in insulin independence for a small number of patients (Goss et al., 2002).

Type 1 diabetes mellitus typically occurs in people 20 years of age and younger. In most cases, onset occurs around age 10 to 12 in girls and age 12 to 14 in boys.

In uncontrolled or untreated type 1 diabetes mellitus, the body cannot use glucose for energy, because little or no insulin is present to deposit glucose into the cells. Therefore, the body starts to break down its fat stores for energy. Although fat has more energy than carbohydrate (glucose), excessive breakdown of fat leads to a buildup of compounds called ketone bodies. The brain and central nervous system can use ketone bodies for energy for a short time, but the buildup of ketone bodies makes the blood more acidic and can result in metabolic *ketoacidosis* (also known as diabetic ketoacidosis), leading to coma and possibly death. (Note that the brain and central nervous system preferentially use glucose for energy.)

People who have uncontrolled type 1 diabetes mellitus have several characteristics: underweight or normal body weight, frequent urination (polyuria), frequent hunger (polyphagia), frequent thirst (polydipsia), hyperglycemia (high levels of blood glucose), and ketotic breath (sweet-smelling breath) (Alberti & Zimmet, 1998).

Type 2 Diabetes Mellitus

With type 2 diabetes mellitus, the pancreas does produce insulin, but the number of insulin receptors may be downregulated, resulting in decreased tissue sensitivity to insulin. Type 2 diabetes mellitus is typically a comorbidity of overweight and obesity. Approximately 90% to 95% of those who have diabetes mellitus in the United States have type 2 diabetes mellitus. Type 2 diabetes mellitus usually occurs after age 45, but because of the increased rate of obesity among all ages, type 2 diabetes mellitus occurs in people of all ages, including young children.

People with type 2 diabetes mellitus can usually manage the disease by losing weight, which they can accomplish through healthy nutrition and exercise. Nonetheless, many people with type 2 diabetes mellitus take oral hypoglycemic agents (for example, Metformin, or glucophage) that help to control their glucose levels. Sometimes, people with type 2 diabetes mellitus also require insulin, but we will not discuss in detail the medications used for type 2 diabetes mellitus.

The signs and symptoms of type 2 diabetes mellitus include some symptoms of type 1 diabetes mellitus (for example, polyuria, polydipsia, polyphagia), as well as repeated infections or skin sores that heal slowly or not at all, overall fatigue, or tingling or numbness in the hands or feet. Symptoms develop more slowly with type 2 diabetes mellitus than they do with type 1 diabetes mellitus. The primary cause of type 2 diabetes mellitus is obesity; most people with type 2 diabetes mellitus are significantly overweight (Alberti & Zimmet, 1998).

Gestational Diabetes Mellitus

Gestational diabetes mellitus is defined as any degree of glucose tolerance with inception or first detection during pregnancy. This definition holds true whether or not insulin or changes to the diet are used for treatment, and whether or not the symptoms persist after pregnancy. Gestational diabetes mellitus complicates about 7% of all pregnancies in the United States (200,000 cases annually). Moderate physical activity has been shown to lower the blood glucose levels in pregnant women. See chapter 4 for more details on safe exercise during pregnancy.

Gestational diabetes mellitus is a condition characterized by high blood glucose levels during pregnancy. It can result from hormonal changes that occur because of pregnancy. If neglected, gestational diabetes mellitus can cause the baby to produce too much insulin and gain too much weight, increasing the risk of premature delivery (Alberti & Zimmet, 1998; Pettitt, 1998).

Typically, blood glucose levels return to normal after birth, but women who contract gestational diabetes mellitus are susceptible to acquiring type 2 diabetes mellitus later in life. See table 7.1 for eating tips for women with gestational diabetes mellitus.

Metabolic Syndrome

Much discussion occurs about the *metabolic syndrome*, yet the definition of this syndrome may not be clear to all. The metabolic syndrome is defined as having several conditions occur together, including obesity, insulin resistance, diabetes or *prediabetes*, hypertension, and high blood lipid levels. According to the Adult Treatment Panel III (ATP III) criteria, a person has the metabolic syndrome if he or she has three or more of the following conditions (Expert Panel on Detection, Evaluation, and Treatment of High Blood Cholesterol in Adults, 2001):

- Abdominal obesity: waist circumference greater than 102 cm (40 in.) in men or greater than 88 cm (35 in.) in women

- Hypertriglyceridemia (high blood triglyceride levels): triglyceride level greater than 150 mg per dl (1.69 mmol per L)

- Low high-density lipoprotein cholesterol (HDL-C) levels: less than 40 mg per dl (1.03 mmol per L) in men or less than 50 mg per dl (1.29 mmol per L) in women

- Hypertension (high blood pressure): greater than 130/85 mmHg

- High fasting blood glucose levels: greater than 110 mg per dl (6.1 mmol per L)

Table 7.1 Nutritional Tips for Women With Gestational Diabetes Mellitus

Tip	Details
Eat three small meals and two or three snacks at consistent times during the day.	Do not skip meals or snacks.
Eat less carbohydrate at breakfast (usually no more than 45 g of carbohydrate); this may vary from one person to another.	Insulin resistance is greatest at this time of day.
Eat consistent amounts of carbohydrate across all meals and smaller amounts consistent across all snacks. Strive to consume the same total amount of carbohydrate each day as well.	The object is to maintain blood glucose levels by being consistent in intake throughout the day, from day to day, and by not skipping meals.
With morning sickness, consume one or two servings of carbohydrate (for example, crackers, pretzels, and so on) before getting out of bed in the morning.	Examples of one serving are 6 crackers, 3 oz of pretzels, 1/2 cup of cereal, and 1 slice of bread.
Consuming high-fiber foods is important.	Ideally, breads, pastas, and other grain products should be whole grain.
Avoid high-sugar and high-fat foods.	
Drink plenty of liquids during the day (about 8 cups of fluid per day).	Avoid sugary drinks and excessive consumption of juices.
Ensure adequate vitamins and minerals in foods eaten.	If even one food group is omitted, consider a general multivitamin and mineral supplement (unless already taking a prenatal vitamin).

From S.L. Volpe, S.B. Sabelawski, and C.R. Mohr, 2007, *Fitness nutrition for special dietary needs* (Champaign, IL: Human Kinetics).

According to the World Health Organization (Alberti & Zimmet, 1998), a person meets the criteria for having the metabolic syndrome if he or she has diagnosed diabetes mellitus, *or* impaired glucose tolerance, *or* impaired (high) fasting glucose levels, *or* insulin resistance, and two or more of the following:

- hypertension (high blood pressure): greater than 160/90 mmHg
- *hyperlipidemia* (high blood triglyceride levels): greater than or equal to 150 mg per dl (1.69 mmol per L)
- low HDL-C levels: less than or equal to 35 mg per dl (0.905 mmol per L) in men or less than or equal to 39 mg per dl (1.01 mmol per L) in women
- central obesity: waist-to-hip ratio greater than 0.90 in men or greater than 0.85 in women *or* a BMI greater than 30 in men or women
- microalbuminuria: urinary excretion rate greater than or equal to 20 g per minute or an albumin-to-creatinine ratio greater than or equal to 20 mg per g

About 24% of the adult population in the United States has metabolic syndrome, and many may not even know it. The data from other regions around the world vary because different definitions of the metabolic syndrome are used. Nonetheless, European studies suggest that between 12% and 25% of the European population has metabolic syndrome, which is similar to the percentage reported in Australia and North America (Laaksonen et al., 2002; Rennie, McCarthy, Yazdgerdi, Marmot, & Brunner, 2003; Sattar et al., 2003; Villegas, Perry, Creagh, Hinchion, & O'Halloran, 2003). Asian countries appear to have lower prevalence of the syndrome (5% to 16% of the population) (Gupta et al., 2003; Lee et al., 2004).

Obviously, a universally acceptable definition of metabolic syndrome is needed. To date, the ATP III and WHO guidelines are used. In general, they focus on the same symptoms. If a person presents with one or more of the previously listed criteria, depending on his or her overall health history and family history, the others should probably be assessed. Regardless of the formal definition of the metabolic syndrome, the best strategy for prevention is physical activity

on most days of the week and maintenance of a healthy body weight.

Prediabetes

Prediabetes is a bit different from the metabolic syndrome. Before contracting type 2 diabetes mellitus, people typically have prediabetes. Prediabetes is characterized by blood glucose levels that are higher than normal yet not high enough to be diagnosed as type 2 diabetes mellitus. Approximately 41 million people in the United States, age 40 to 74, have prediabetes. Prediabetes may start to damage the circulatory system, although it is not considered full-blown diabetes mellitus (www.diabetes.org/pre-diabetes.jsp).

Those who should be screened for prediabetes include overweight adults age 45 and older and those under age 45 who are significantly overweight and have one or more of the following:

- Family history of diabetes mellitus
- Low HDL-C and high triglyceride levels
- Hypertension
- Previously diagnosed impaired glucose tolerance or impaired (high) fasting glucose levels
- History of gestational diabetes or giving birth to a baby weighing more than 9 lb (4.1 kg)

If people work to control blood glucose levels when they have prediabetes, type 2 diabetes mellitus may be delayed or may never even occur (www.diabetes.org/pre-diabetes.jsp). The National Institute of Diabetes and Digestive and Kidney Diseases and the American Diabetes Association published a position statement titled "The Prevention or Delay of Type 2 Diabetes." Health care professionals can use this position statement in treating people with prediabetes (www.diabetes.org/pre-diabetes.jsp).

Prediabetes (and hence, diabetes mellitus) can occur in people of all ages and races. Nonetheless, some groups are at higher risk for contracting the disease than others. Prediabetes and diabetes mellitus are more widespread in older persons, as well as in African Americans, Latinos, Native Americans, Asian Americans, and Pacific Islanders (www.diabetes.org/pre-diabetes.jsp).

The primary tests used to determine prediabetes are fasting plasma (blood) glucose test

(FPG or FBG) or the oral glucose tolerance test (OGTT). FPG is simply an assessment of blood glucose levels when a person has fasted. The OGTT is measured both at fasting and then at 1 and 2 hours after consumption of a sugary beverage (typically, 50 g of a glucose beverage). The OGTT allows the clinician to assess how quickly a person's body can remove the excess glucose from the blood and bring it into the tissues. If FPG levels are high, the person has impaired fasting glucose (IFG). If blood glucose levels are high after the OGTT, the person is diagnosed as having impaired glucose tolerance (IGT) (www. diabetes.org/pre-diabetes.jsp). See figure 7.1 for normal, prediabetes, and diabetes FPG and OGTT levels.

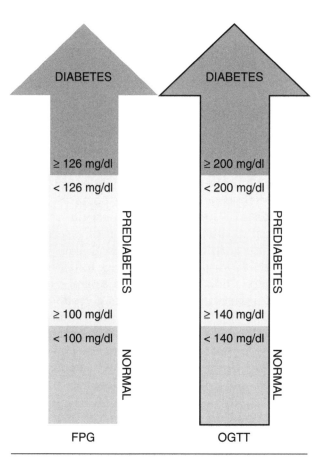

Figure 7.1   Blood glucose levels following a fasting plasma glucose (FPG) and an oral glucose tolerance test (OGTT). These levels diagnose whether a person has normal glucose levels, prediabetes, or diabetes mellitus.

© 2007 American Diabetes Association. From www.diabetes.org. Reprinted with permission from *The American Diabetes Association*.

Polycystic Ovary Syndrome

About 5% of women in the United Sates suffer from *polycystic ovary syndrome* **(PCOS).** PCOS frequently results in obesity, large muscles, large bones, facial hair, male-pattern baldness, acne, and irregular menses (www.drmirkin.com/women/8124.htm). Although not always considered in the diabetes arena, PCOS is closely tied to blood glucose levels. People with PCOS often have insulin resistance or impaired glucose tolerance. Medications and nutrition regimens used for diabetes mellitus treatment may help women with PCOS in the prevention of diabetes, heart disease, and obesity. If a woman thinks that she may have PCOS, she should obtain a sonogram of her ovaries and then seek appropriate medical treatment.

Complications of Diabetes Mellitus

Left untreated, diabetes mellitus can result in life-threatening complications, including neuropathy (disease of the nervous system), angiopathy (cardiovascular disease), retinopathy (disease of the eyes that could lead to blindness), and nephropathy (disease of the kidneys that could lead to kidney failure). Neuropathy can cause loss of sense of feeling, which often leads to wounds that never heal because the person with diabetes mellitus does not feel them. Amputations of the lower limbs can result if these infections become so severe that they result in gangrene and other complications. Diabetes mellitus is the leading cause of new blindness in people 20 to 74 years of age. In addition, 40% of new cases of renal disease result from diabetes mellitus. Although these long-term diseases can occur in all people, those with diabetes mellitus have a greater risk of contracting the chronic conditions described earlier. Also, as noted earlier, if blood glucose levels are not controlled, metabolic (or diabetic) ketoacidosis could occur (Alberti & Zimmet, 1998).

NUTRITION

In general, people with diabetes mellitus should consume meals and snacks at regular intervals each day. This practice will help maintain blood glucose levels within normal limits and prevent large swings in blood glucose. A person with diabetes mellitus should consume a simple carbohydrate if his or her blood glucose level is less than 100 mg per dl (5.56 mmol per L). A simple sugar will easily be absorbed and will help increase the blood glucose level. People with diabetes mellitus should carry high-carbohydrate foods with them all the time—while exercising, when in the car, and at work or play. A person with diabetes mellitus can carry a tube of icing to ensure that he or she can obtain sugar quickly, if need be. Icing in a tube is shelf stable. A person with diabetes mellitus who is suffering from hypoglycemia can simply place it between the cheek and gums. Chewing or swallowing would not be necessary. Glucose tablets and orange juice are other options. A person who exercises and has diabetes mellitus should consume complex carbohydrates throughout the day to maintain blood glucose levels and maintain glycogen stores for exercise.

Carbohydrate Intake Before, During, and After Exercise

Carbohydrate intake is important for all athletes, those with and without diabetes, to fill and maintain glycogen stores for energy during exercise. People with diabetes, however, need to focus on their carbohydrate intake even more because they do not want to become hypoglycemic during exercise. Active people with diabetes should consume about 8 to 10 g of carbohydrate per kg of body weight per day (about 3.5 to 4.5 g of carbohydrate per lb of body weight) (Colberg, 2001), the same amount recommended for athletes who do not have diabetes. This quantity is a guideline that applies to those who exercise for a minimum of 45 minutes per day. Those who exercise regularly for less than 45 minutes per day may want to adjust carbohydrate intake to about 6 to 8 g of carbohydrate per kg of body weight per day (approximately 2.7 to 3.6 g of carbohydrate per lb of body weight).

These guidelines need to be tailored to each person, because everyone is unique. In general, those with diabetes mellitus should spread their carbohydrate intake evenly throughout the day to ensure that the body maintains a consistent amount of glucose in the blood. Carbohydrate can be consumed before, during, and after exercise, but blood glucose concentrations must be assessed daily to ascertain changes in blood glu-

cose levels surrounding the exercise bout. Those who exercise longer than 30 to 60 minutes may need to consume carbohydrate during exercise to ensure that they maintain blood glucose levels. By self-monitoring blood glucose, the person with diabetes mellitus will know how much carbohydrate will be required. Research suggests that blood glucose concentrations should remain between 70 and 150 mg per dl (3.9 and 8.3 mmol per L) for optimal performance (Walsh & Roberts, 1994).

The type of carbohydrate is also important. Complex whole grains are better choices than simple carbohydrates. Complex carbohydrates provide sustained energy, and whole-grain products provide more nutrients and fiber. Fiber may help control blood glucose levels. For a summary guide to diabetic carbohydrate consumption, see the section *"Guidelines for Carbohydrate Intake for Active People With Diabetes."*

Some evidence suggests that consuming foods with a high glycemic index within 30 minutes after exercise may help replenish glycogen stores. But some controversy still exists about this recommendation. Glycemic index refers to the increase in blood glucose that occurs after consumption of a certain food. Glycemic index is assessed by having a person ingest about 50 g of a carbohydrate food. Blood glucose is measured over a 2-hour period. Glycemic index values for different foods are calculated by comparing measurements of their effect on blood glucose with an equal carbohydrate portion of a reference food. The current method uses glucose as the reference food, giving it a glycemic index value of 100 by definition. If, for example, a person ingests 50 g of a particular food and its glycemic index is 80%, eating that particular food results in a rise of blood glucose that is 80% as great as the increase following the consumption of pure glucose. Nonetheless, several factors can affect the glycemic index of a food, including the structure of the carbohydrate, its absorption rate, the time of consumption of the carbohydrate, the types of foods consumed previously, other substances within the food (for example, protein and fat), and individual differences in body chemistry.

Lower glycemic index foods consumed 30 to 60 minutes before a workout or competition may be beneficial because little or no drop in blood glucose would occur, which could lead to a higher concentration of fat in the blood to be used for energy. The available energy in the blood could spare muscle glycogen, leading to better performance and less fatigue. As stated earlier, some evidence suggests that consuming high glycemic index foods after exercise might help promote muscle glycogen storage, but experts disagree about the effect of glycemic index on performance. This issue is especially controversial in regard to athletes who have diabetes. Athletes should experiment with foods of different glycemic indexes during practice, not during competition.

As noted earlier, because of individual chemical makeup, foods with a high glycemic index may not elicit the same increase in blood glucose in all athletes and may result in greater increases in athletes with diabetes mellitus compared with athletes without diabetes mellitus. Table 7.2 lists some foods that have high, moderate, and low glycemic indexes. To obtain information on the glycemic index of more foods, we refer the reader to the following Web site: www.glycemicindex.com.

Preventing Low Blood Glucoses During Exercise

Moderate to intense activity may cause blood glucose levels to decrease for the 24 hours after exercise. Sometimes referred to as the lag effect of exercise, this effect of exercise can be positive, but blood glucose must be monitored closely before and after exercise, as well as throughout the day, to avoid hypoglycemia.

If blood glucose levels are less than 100 mg per dl (5.56 mmol per L) immediately after exercise,

Table 7.2   Glycemic Indexes of Different Foods

High glycemic index foods (>70%)	Moderate glycemic index foods (56% to 69%)	Low glycemic index foods (<55%)
Waffles	New potatoes	Al dente (firm) pasta
White bagel or bread	Popcorn	Peas
Corn flakes	Canned kidney beans	Skim milk
Graham crackers	Corn	Barley
Parsnips	Brown rice	Chickpeas
Rutabaga	Oatmeal	Lentils
Soda crackers	Rye bread	Baked beans
Baked white potato	Whole-wheat bread	Plum
Watermelon	Pineapple	Orange
Hard candy	Raisins	Plain yogurt
Honey	Overripe banana	Underripe banana
Jellybeans	Grapes	Apple
Doughnut	Angel food cake	Soy milk
Wafer biscuits	Unsweetened muffin	Whole-grain breads
Rice cakes	Mangoes	Meat-filled ravioli
Broad beans	Table sugar	Peanuts
Gatorade	Orange juice	Grapefruit

Note: Because metabolism varies somewhat from person to person, some people may have a response to some foods that gives those items a higher glycemic index than those indicated in the columns. Nevertheless, this table provides a good general guideline for high, moderate, and low glycemic index foods.

From S.L. Volpe, S.B. Sabelawski, and C.R. Mohr, 2007, *Fitness nutrition for special dietary needs* (Champaign, IL: Human Kinetics).

Guidelines for Carbohydrate Intake
for Active People With Diabetes

- Include carbohydrate from a variety of whole grains, fruits, vegetables, and skim milk.
- Complex carbohydrates are especially important because they are good sources of fiber, which delays the absorption of sugar into the bloodstream (as well as helps to control weight).
- Consume approximately 8 to 10 g of carbohydrate per kg of body weight (about 3.5 to 4.5 g of carbohydrate per lb of body weight) every day. This amount is the same as that recommended for those without diabetes.
- Avoid low-carbohydrate diets that restrict total carbohydrate intake to less than 130 g per day because such diets may affect blood lipids negatively.
- Be consistent with carbohydrate intake.
- Use nonnutritive sweetener safely by remaining within the Acceptable Daily Intakes (ADI) established by the FDA.

Polyols and Novel Sugar Sweeteners

Type	Kcal/g	Regulatory status	Other names	Estimated Daily Intake (EDI) or Acceptable Daily Intake (ADI)	Description
MONOSACCHARIDE POLYOLS OR NOVEL SUGARS					
Sorbitol	2.6	GRAS*–Label must warn about a laxative effect	Same as chemical name		50-70% as sweet as sucrose; some individuals experience a laxative effect from a load of 50 g.
Mannitol	1.6	Approved food additive; the label must warn about a laxative effect	Same as chemical name		50-70% as sweet as sucrose; some individuals experience a laxative effect from a load of 20 g.
Xylitol	2.4	Approved food additive for use in foods for special dietary needs	Same as chemical name		As sweet as sucrose; new forms have better free-flowing abilities.
Erythritol	0.2	Independent GRAS determinations; no questions from FDA	Same as chemical name	EDI mean: 1 g/p/d; 90th percentile: 4 g/p/d	60-80% as sweet as sucrose; also acts as a flavor enhancer, formulation aid, humectant, stabilizer and thickener, sequestrant, and texturizer.
D-Tagatose	1.5	Independent GRAS determinations; no questions from FDA	Same as chemical name	EDI mean: 7.5 g/p/d; 90th percentile: 14 g/p/d ADI 15 grams/60 kg adult/d	75-92% as sweet as sucrose; sweetness synegizer, functions also as a texturizer, stabilizer, humectant, and formulation aid.
DISACCHARIDE POLYOLS OR NOVEL SUGARS					
Isomalt	2	GRAS affirmation petition filed	Same as chemical name		45-65% as sweet as sucrose; used as a bulking agent.

Type	Kcal/g	Regulatory status	Other names	Estimated Daily Intake (EDI) or Acceptable Daily Intake (ADI)	Description
DISACCHARIDE POLYOLS OR NOVEL SUGARS *(cont'd)*					
Lactitol	2	GRAS affirmation petition filed	Same as chemical name		30-40% as sweet as sucrose; used as a bulking agent.
Maltitol	2.1	GRAS affirmation petition filed	Same as chemical name		90% as sweet as sucrose; used as a bulking agent.
Trehalose	4	Independent GRAS determinations; no questions from FDA	Same as chemical name	EDI mean: 34 g/p/d; 90th percentile: 68 g/p/d	45% as sweet as sucrose; functions also as a texturizer, stabilizer, and humectant.
POLY-SACCHARIDE POLYOLS					
HSH	3	GRAS affirmation petition filed	Hydrogenated starch hydrolysates; maltitol syrup		25-50% as sweet as sucrose (depending on the monosaccharide composition).

*GRAS = Generally recognized as safe.
From S.L. Volpe, S.B. Sabelawski, and C.R. Mohr, 2007, *Fitness nutrition for special dietary needs* (Champaign, IL: Human Kinetics). Adapted from position of the American Dietetic Association: Use of Nutritive and Nonnutritive Sweeteners. *J Am Diet Assoc.* 2004; 104:255-275.

Approved Nonnutritive Sweeteners

Type	Kcal/g	Regulatory status	Other names	Description
Saccharin	0	Approved as a sweetener for beverages and as a tabletop sweetener in foods with specific maximum amounts allowed	Sweet and Low, Sweet Twin, Sweet N' Low Brown, Necta Sweet, Sugar Twin	200-700 times sweeter than sucrose; noncariogenic and produces no glycemic response; synergizes the sweetening power of nutritive and nonnutritive sweeteners; sweetening power is not reduced with heating
Aspartame	4*	Approved as a general purpose sweetener	Nutrasweet, Equal	160-220 times sweeter than sucrose; noncariogenic and produces limited glycemic response
Acesulfame	0	Approved as a general purpose sweetener	Sunett, Sweet & Safe, Sweet One	200 times sweeter than sucrose; noncariogenic and produces no glycemic response; synergizes the sweetening power of nutritive and nonnutritive sweeteners; is not reduced with heating
Sucralose	0	Approved as a general purpose sweetener	Splenda	600 times sweeter than sucrose; noncariogenic and produces no glycemic response; sweetening power is not reduced with heating
Neotame	0	Approved as a general purpose sweetener	Not available at time of publication	8,000 times sweeter than sucrose; noncariogenic and produces no glycemic response; sweetening power is not reduced with heating

*This sweetener does provide energy; however, because of the intense sweetness, the amount of energy derived from it is negligible.
From S.L. Volpe, S.B. Sabelawski, and C.R. Mohr, 2007, *Fitness nutrition for special dietary needs* (Champaign, IL: Human Kinetics). Adapted from position of the American Dietetic Association: Use of Nutritive and Nonnutritive Sweeteners. *J Am Diet Assoc.* 2004; 104:255-275.

the person can do one or more of the following to prevent this from occurring in the future:

- Increase carbohydrate intake before exercise.
- Decrease the dose of insulin for the next exercise session.
- Consider decreasing the insulin dosage following exercise.
- If blood glucose levels at bedtime are still less than 100 mg per dl (5.56 mmol per L), increase the evening snack, perhaps even double it, ensure that the snack contains a mixture of carbohydrate and protein, and be sure to be properly hydrated.

The major goal is to prevent hypoglycemia as a result of exercise. To prevent postexercise hypoglycemia, here are some specific recommendations:

- Consume 15 g of carbohydrate if not planning to eat in the 30 to 60 minutes before exercise (for example, 1 cup of puffed wheat cereal with 1/2 cup of skim milk).
- Take in 15 g of carbohydrate and 7 g of protein if not planning to eat for more than 60 minutes before exercise (for example, two slices of whole-wheat bread with 1 tbsp of peanut butter).

These recommendations apply only if a person does not have much time to eat before exercising. We recommend that a person with diabetes mellitus consume a high-carbohydrate snack with fluids before exercise to avoid hypoglycemia and any dangers that can occur if he or she becomes hypoglycemic during exercise.

Exchange List for Meal Planning and Carbohydrate Counting

The Exchange List for Meal Planning (developed jointly by the American Diabetes Association and the American Dietetic Association) and Carbohydrate Counting are two ways to ensure that a person who has either type 1 or type 2 diabetes mellitus consumes a consistent amount of food, namely carbohydrates, throughout the day, which will lead to better glucose control. Both methods aim to spread the amount of carbohydrate (and fat and protein) evenly throughout the day and help the person with diabetes mellitus

Myths About Athletes and Diabetes Mellitus

Before people became aware that many successful athletes had diabetes mellitus, individuals with diabetes mellitus were often discouraged from playing sports. Blood glucose control was the biggest issue, of course. But it was thought that if a person with diabetes mellitus became injured, the healing process would take so long that if the person had even a slight form of neuropathy, gangrene could develop. As more people with diabetes mellitus became physically active and as more professional athletes with diabetes mellitus discussed their disease, professionals in these fields developed better nutrition and exercise guidelines. The guest dietitian in this chapter provides an excellent case study of a professional football player who was diagnosed with type 1 diabetes mellitus.

Some Famous Athletes With Diabetes Mellitus

Arthur Ashe (professional tennis player)

Ayden Byle (first person with type 1 diabetes mellitus to run across North America)

Bobby Clarke (professional ice hockey player)

Ty Cobb (professional baseball player)

Scott Coleman (first man with diabetes mellitus to swim across the English Channel)

James "Buster" Douglas (boxing)

Kenny Duckett (professional football player)

Chris Dudley (professional basketball player)

Ned Edwards (squash)

Pam Fernandes (Para-Olympian)

Curt Fraiser (professional hockey player)

"Smokin' Joe" Fraizer (professional boxer)

Bill Gullickson (professional baseball player)

Gary Hall (Olympic swimmer, gold medalist)

Jonathon Hayes (professional football player)

Catfish Hunter (professional baseball player)

Jason Johnson (professional baseball player)

Adapted from www.angelarose.com/FamousDiabetics/FamSports.htm.

keep regular eating habits. Again, the main goal is to control blood glucose levels. These methods can be extremely helpful for people with diabetes mellitus who exercise, especially after they establish a consistent exercise routine. For more information, visit the American Diabetes Association Web site at www.diabetes.org.

Low-Carbohydrate Diets

Low-carbohydrate diets have become increasingly popular over the last several years, despite the fact that the Atkins diet has been around since the 1970s. Because they require a person to restrict intake of certain foods or food groups, in this case carbohydrate, low-carbohydrate, high-protein diets are considered a type of fad diet. Carbohydrate intake is typically limited to 20 g or less per day in the early stages of the diet. It then increases to 60 g per day for weight-loss regimen and to 95 g per day for maintenance. The goal of high-protein diets is to increase ketone production in the body, which is supposed to decrease appetite. The negative effect of high **ketone bodies** is that although they can be used for energy early on, they will not be able to sustain the energy needed by the brain and central nervous system (which preferentially use glucose, or blood sugar, for energy) for a long period. Subsequently, ketoacidosis can occur, which can lead to a coma. In a person with diabetes, who already is at greater risk of having this occur, the high-protein diet could be a double-edged sword.

High-protein diets allow unlimited consumption of meat, a high-fat food. High-protein diets limit fruits, vegetables, and grains, foods that protect against heart disease and cancer. The high intake of meat (animal fat and cholesterol) could lead to heart disease, cancer, **gout**, kidney stones, hypertension, and the like.

Although weight loss has been reported in those who consume low-carbohydrate diets, long-term studies have not found differences in 1-year follow-ups between low-carbohydrate, high-protein diets and higher-carbohydrate, low-fat diets (Foster et al., 2003). Furthermore, weight loss typically occurs because of the limited food choices and the higher fat intake (greater satiety) in high-protein diets.

A higher-protein, lower-carbohydrate diet may in fact be beneficial for people with diabetes mellitus, but not with carbohydrate intake as low as that promoted in the Atkins diet and others. A person with diabetes mellitus may benefit from better glucose control if he or she consumes a diet with about 45% or 50% of total energy intake from carbohydrate (complex, whole grains), about 20% of total energy intake from protein, and about 30% of total energy intake from mostly monounsaturated fats (for example, olive oil, canola oil, and avocados). Not all researchers have reported positive results with glucose control from high-protein diets; thus more research is required (Sargrad, Homko, Mozzoli, & Boden, 2005). Our recommendation is for people with diabetes to reduce carbohydrate intake slightly from the average intake of 55% to 60% of total energy from carbohydrate to a more moderate intake of 45% to 50% of total energy from carbohydrate. This recommendation varies significantly from the extreme low-carbohydrate, high-protein intake advocated by the Atkins diet and others.

Another concern of high-protein diets is that they provide a limited amount of vitamins and minerals because of the emphasis on consuming less fruits and vegetables. Again, a diet with a modified carbohydrate intake would still encourage fruit and vegetable consumption. Certainly, people with diabetes mellitus must watch the amount of simple sugars that they consume, including those from fruits, but by spreading the intake of fruits throughout the day, they can maintain blood glucose levels and obtain the antioxidant and fiber benefits from fruits and vegetables.

PHYSICAL ACTIVITY

For people with diabetes mellitus, nutrition and a sound exercise program are the cornerstones of maintaining a healthy body weight and healthy blood glucose levels. Exercise is important to those with either type 2 diabetes mellitus or type 1 diabetes mellitus to help control blood glucose concentrations, maintain a healthy body weight, and prevent long-term complications from occurring.

Importance of Exercise for People With Diabetes Mellitus

Exercise may even "cure" people of prediabetes, the metabolic syndrome, and type 2 diabetes mellitus. Regular exercise helps maintain glucose

Sample Meal Plan for People
With Type 1 and Type 2 Diabetes Mellitus

This sample meal plan provides a healthy variety of nutrients, food choices, vitamins, and minerals. The registered dietitian must work with each client individually to determine what may work for that person. In this case, the type of diabetes mellitus will play a role, as will the person's likes and dislikes, allergies, gender, age, culture, and so forth.

Breakfast
- 1/2 cup of bran cereal = 113 g
- 1/2 cup of skim milk = 120 ml
- 1/2 medium banana = 40 g
- 1 cup of coffee = 240 ml
- 1 packet of nonnutritive sweetener = 5 g

Snack
- 1/2 cup of cottage cheese = 120 g
- 1 medium pear = 80 g
- 8 oz of water = 240 ml

Lunch
- Tuna salad sandwich
  - 2 oz of tuna salad = 57 g
  - 2 slices of multigrain bread = 80 g
  - 2 slices each of lettuce and tomato = 40 g
- 1 cup of vegetable soup = 240 ml
- 8 oz of Crystal Light beverage = 240 ml

Snack
- 1/2 whole-wheat bagel = 40 g
- 2 tbsp of peanut butter = 30 g
- 1/2 cup of fresh fruit = 113 g
- 8 oz of water = 240 ml

Dinner
- 3 oz of baked chicken breast = 90 g
- 2 small baked red potatoes = 50 g
- 1/2 cup of steamed carrots = 115 g
- 1/2 cup of steamed fresh green beans = 115 g
- 2 tsp of butter or margarine = 10 g
- 8 oz of skim milk = 240 ml

Snack
- 4 oz of low-fat vanilla yogurt = 113 g
- 1/2 cup of mixed berries (blueberries, blackberries, raspberries) = 113 g
- 3 squares of graham crackers = 30 g
- 8 oz of water or Crystal Light beverage = 240 ml

This sample meal plan provides at least 100% of the Dietary Reference Intakes (DRIs) for energy, protein, fiber, vitamins A, C, E, B_6, B_{12}, thiamin, riboflavin, niacin, folate, calcium, iron, magnesium, phosphorus, zinc, and approximately

- 2,000 kcal (8,360 kJ),
- 104 g of protein,
- 60 g of fat,
- 30 g of fiber, and
- 3,600 mg of sodium.

Sample Meal Plan for Women With Gestational Diabetes Mellitus

Breakfast
- 1 hard-boiled egg = 45 g
- 2 slices of whole-wheat toast = 80 g
- 1 tsp margarine = 5 g
- 4 oz of orange juice = 120 ml

Snack
- 1 cup of Raisin Bran cereal = 226 g
- 1 cup of skim milk = 240 ml
- 1 oz of sunflower seeds = 28 g
- 1 medium banana = 80 g
- 8 oz of water = 240 ml

Lunch
- Cheese sandwich
- 1 oz of low-fat cheese = 28 g
- 2 slices of whole-grain bread = 80 g
- 2 cups of mixed greens salad = 460 g
- 1 tbsp of vinaigrette dressing = 15 g
- 1 cup of skim milk = 240 ml

Snack
- 1/2 cup of mixed nuts = 120 g
- 1 cup of fresh watermelon = 80 g
- 8 oz of water = 240 ml

Dinner

- 3 oz of baked pork chops = 90 g
- 1 cup of brown rice = 120 g
- 1 cup of steamed asparagus = 113 g
- 1 tbsp of olive oil for the asparagus = 15 g
- 1/2 cup of applesauce = 113 g
- 1 cup of skim milk = 240 ml

Snack

- 1 cup of low-fat vanilla yogurt = 230 g
- 3/4 cup of Grape Nuts cereal = 170 g
- 1 cup of fresh strawberries = 113 g
- 8 oz of water = 240 ml

This sample meal plan provides at least 100% of the Dietary Reference Intakes (DRIs) for energy, protein, fiber, vitamins A, C, E, B_6, B_{12}, thiamin, riboflavin, niacin, folate, calcium, iron, magnesium, phosphorus, zinc, and approximately

- 2,500 kcal (10,450 kJ),
- 115 g of protein,
- 90 g of fat,
- 41 g of fiber, and
- 4,200 mg of sodium.

From S.L. Volpe, S.B. Sabelawski, and C.R. Mohr, 2007, *Fitness nutrition for special dietary needs* (Champaign, IL: Human Kinetics).

control (especially long-term control of glycosylated hemoglobin levels in the blood) and can help prevent long-term complications resulting from diabetes (American Diabetes Association, 2004; Boule, Haddard, Kenny, Wells, & Sigal, 2001; Hu et al., 1991). Measurement of glycosylated hemoglobin (HbA1c), typically done every 3 months, assesses long-term glucose control. Some glucose is always bound to hemoglobin, even in people without diabetes. Over the long term, however, if a person with diabetes has not controlled his or her blood glucose, this measurement will be higher than normal and will indicate that the person does not have good adherence to his or her diet, exercise regimen, or medication.

As with other people, regular exercise results in cardiovascular disease prevention for those with diabetes mellitus. Because they have a greater risk of cardiovascular disease, exercise is especially important for people with diabetes mellitus. Exercise helps decrease risk of cardiovascular disease by reducing lipid levels, decreasing blood pressure, and maintaining or decreasing body weight (Horton, 1998). The reduction in body weight is directly related to improvement in insulin sensitivity. In addition, exercise increases the production of a protein called GLUT4, which helps potentiate insulin, thereby resulting in improved insulin sensitivity in those with type 2 diabetes mellitus. Among people with type 1 diabetes mellitus, improved sensitivity will reduce the amount of insulin required. Note that for people with either type 1 or type 2 diabetes mellitus, as well as other types of diabetes mellitus, prediabetes, and metabolic

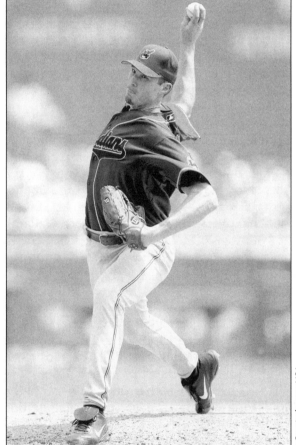

© Sportschrome USA

When Jason Johnson was diagnosed with type 1 diabetes at age 11, he was afraid he wouldn't be able to continue playing baseball, a game he loved above all others. His physician told him to work hard and take care of his diabetes. Taking good care of his health, Jason wasn't limited by his diabetes. Here he pitches a winning game for the Cleveland Indians against the Detroit Tigers in 2006.

syndrome, daily exercise is important in maintaining stable blood glucose and HbA1c levels (Schneider, Khachadurian, Amorosa, Clemow, & Ruderman, 1992). Of course, exercising from 3 to 5 days a week is better than no exercise, but people need to be encouraged to exercise daily for blood glucose maintenance and prevention of hypoglycemia, especially those with type 1 diabetes mellitus. If a person does not exercise daily, insulin and meal planning will need to be adjusted.

Contraindications to Exercise for People With Diabetes Mellitus

Despite the benefits of exercise for people with diabetes mellitus, there are contraindications to exercising. If a person's blood glucose (sugar) levels are greater than 250 mg per dl and ketones are present in the urine (ketonuria), the person should not exercise. He or she should use caution with exercise if ketones are not present and blood glucose levels are greater then 300 mg per dl. Further dehydration (with exercise) and ketone body buildup can result in ketoacidosis.

In people with type 1 diabetes mellitus, ketonuria indicates a lack of insulin and the immediate need for an insulin injection. Exercise at this time would produce more ketone bodies and thus put this person in danger of metabolic (or diabetic) ketoacidosis, as well as hypoglycemia. Keep in mind that the symptoms of *ketosis* are similar to the symptoms of metabolic ketoacidosis. Ketosis, however, is a condition that occurs when the diet is low in carbohydrate and glycogen stores are depleted. The body must then rely primarily on fat and protein as a fuel. Ketosis, therefore, is the condition of having higher than normal levels of ketones in the blood and urine. If this condition worsens, metabolic (diabetic) ketoacidosis can occur. Metabolic (diabetic) ketoacidosis, basically a severe ketosis that causes the pH of the blood to drop below 7.4, is a medical condition typically caused by uncontrolled diabetes mellitus, hyperglycemia, ketonuria, and increased levels of the hormone glucagon (which acts to increase blood glucose levels when they are low in the blood).

People with diabetes mellitus should be screened thoroughly before beginning any exercise program. They should be checked for the presence of macrovascular or microvascular complications that may hinder the exercise program because of poor circulation. A medical history, including a thorough physical exam with emphasis on heart function, blood vessel function, vision, kidneys, and nervous system, should be conducted to determine the appropriate exercise prescription.

Exercising With Diabetes Mellitus

Although exercising is imperative to living healthfully with diabetes, the person with diabetes mellitus must speak to his or her physician before starting any exercise regimen to assure that there are no contraindications to exercise. In addition, when a person with diabetes mellitus begins an exercise program, the physician will usually have to adjust the person's insulin and oral hypoglycemic agents.

• **Type I diabetes mellitus**. Although regular exercise is extremely important to people with type 1 diabetes mellitus, blood glucose may decrease during exercise and subsequently increase after exercise. Either may cause rapid development of ketosis, even in people with well-controlled diabetes mellitus. The risk of hypoglycemia during exercise and hyperglycemia after exercise in people with type 1 diabetes mellitus may make participation in sports difficult, either recreationally or competitively. But exercise is not a contraindication to all people with type 1 diabetes mellitus. Thus, we recommend that all people with type 1 diabetes mellitus be evaluated by a physician before beginning an exercise program. They should continue to monitor their blood glucose levels, regularly see their physician for adjustments in their insulin, and consult with their dietitian for adjustments in food intake, especially in the early stages of the exercise program.

• **Type 2 diabetes mellitus**. Regular exercise is extremely important for the treatment of type 2 diabetes mellitus and should be prescribed along with a healthy diet and oral hypoglycemic agents (if medications are needed, although a healthy diet and regular exercise can "cure" type 2 diabetes mellitus). Monitoring blood glucose levels is as important for people with type 2 diabetes mellitus as it is for individuals with type 1 diabetes mellitus. Many people with type 2 diabetes mellitus are obese and may have other complications. Again, people should have a thorough physical examination before beginning

Principles of Prescribing

Based on the results of experimental measurements, the following algorithm has been designed for prescribing exercise to people with diabetes: appropriate motivation, determination of the type of exercise, determination of the intensity of exercise, determination of the duration of exercise, and consideration of related contraindications and complications (Rybka, 1987).

an exercise program. After gaining the approval of his or her physician, a person with type 2 diabetes mellitus can start simply by walking or doing other familiar activities. Multiple bouts of physical activity throughout the day can be beneficial for weight loss, cardiovascular fitness (Jakicic, Winters, Lang, & Wing, 1999), and adherence. Beginning slowly with familiar exercises will increase adherence and decrease the risk of injuries and hypoglycemia.

Tips for Optimal Exercise Conditions

When providing general exercise regimens, several intricacies are of note. Some people with diabetes mellitus exercise regularly. Indeed, many elite athletes have diabetes mellitus. Therefore, a recommendation for a general 30-minute bout of exercise will not be appropriate for the elite athlete with diabetes mellitus. If a person is involved in a long endurance event, for example, he or she will require further instruction about how to monitor blood glucose levels throughout the event to prevent hypoglycemia, dehydration, and so on from occurring. Again, advice must be tailored individually to a person who exercises, based on his or her exercise program, goals, disease state, and so on. This book provides general guidelines that will need to be refined for each person.

• **Longer exercise bouts**. People with either type 1 or type 2 diabetes mellitus who exercise in endurance events such as triathlons or marathons will need to increase their food intake significantly and adjust their insulin and oral hypoglycemic agents (if they are taking them

for type 2 diabetes mellitus). Some individuals with type 1 or type 2 diabetes mellitus have competed in endurance and ultraendurance events or competitively in professional and collegiate sports. These athletes must carefully monitor their energy intake and glucose levels. They should carry some quick-acting carbohydrates with them during their events to maintain blood glucose levels. Many quick-acting carbohydrates are available, including gels, hard candies, carbohydrate-based beverages, sports bars, icing in a tube, and glucose tablets. By following the carbohydrate guidelines outlined earlier in the chapter and monitoring blood glucose concentrations before, during (at least initially), and after each activity, the person with diabetes mellitus who exercises will be able to perform at his or her optimal level. In addition, the athlete with diabetes mellitus and the registered dietitian should be in close contact with the athlete's physician.

• **Blood glucose monitoring**. Blood glucose can either increase or decrease postexercise. As a result of exercise, the liver releases more sugar than usual because during exercise the muscle needs more glucose to supply energy. If insulin in the body is insufficient to control blood glucose levels, blood glucose can increase. This increase can occur immediately after exercise when not enough insulin is available for muscles to take up blood glucose. This circumstance is more typical with type 1 than type 2 diabetes mellitus. Exercise is not recommended if blood glucose levels are less than 100 mg per dl (5.56 mmol per L) or greater than 250 mg per dl (13.9 mmol per L) and urinary ketones are present. Exercise is also contraindicated if blood glucose is greater than 300 mg per dl (16.7 mmol per L) with no ketone bodies present in the urine (for type 1 diabetes mellitus). Exercise is not recommended for those with type 2 diabetes mellitus when blood glucose levels are greater than 400 mg per dl (22.2 mmol per L) and no urinary ketones are present. The major goal is to maintain normal blood glucose levels (70 to 120 mg per dl, or 3.9 to 6.7 mmol per L) before, during, and after exercise. The closer a person with diabetes mellitus can come to maintaining normal blood glucose levels, the less likely it is that he or she will suffer from long-term complications of diabetes, from hypoglycemia during exercise, or from hyperglycemia after exercise. Self-monitoring of blood glucose is crucial to ensuring maintenance of blood glucose levels.

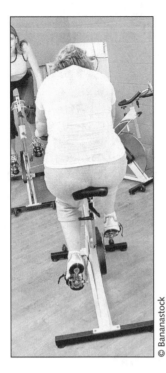

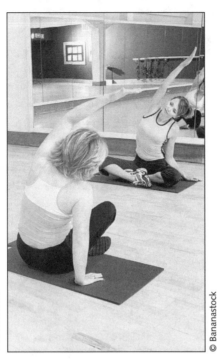

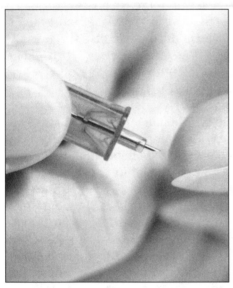

For people with type 1 or type 2 diabetes mellitus, a regular exercise program is essential to maintaining a steady blood glucose concentration and body weight (especially in the case of type 2 diabetes mellitus). Besides engaging in a regular exercise routine and meeting nutritional needs, the person with diabetes mellitus must closely monitor his or her blood glucose levels before and after exercise to facilitate possible adjustments to medications or eating patterns.

- **Hydration**. Hydration is important, especially in the heat, because hydration status can adversely affect blood glucose levels and heart function. Thus, people with diabetes mellitus who exercise must stay properly hydrated. For guidelines on hydration and fluid intake, refer to chapter 1.

- **Other tips**. Like all people who exercise, a person with diabetes mellitus should warm up for the activity in which he or she will participate (at a lower heart rate) and cool down afterward (with stretching). Dressing appropriately is also important. Because neuropathy is a long-term

complication of diabetes mellitus, wearing comfortable, well-fitting socks and good shoes to minimize foot trauma is important. The socks should be comfortable and breathable.

CASE STUDY

Our guest dietitian in this chapter has experience working with a variety of athletes, including those with diabetes mellitus. This case involved a professional football player with type 1 diabetes mellitus. This athlete's body weight and age made him more likely to be diagnosed with type 1 rather than type 2 diabetes mellitus.

K.S. is a 25-year-old, 6 ft 3 in. (190.5 cm), 319 lb (145 kg), 3rd-year offensive lineman for an NFL team. A number one draft pick, he had a great rookie season, and expectations for his 2nd year were high. One week before training camp, he called the team physician to say that he had not been feeling well and had lost weight from his typical 320 lb (145 kg) to 300 lb (126 kg) over 4 weeks. The player complained of weakness and excessive thirst and urination. The team physician advised him to fly in early to be evaluated. The player preferred to drive, and over the 2-day drive north, he made 20 rest stops to urinate. When he arrived at the physician's office, he had blurred vision, headaches, felt nauseated, and was weak. His blood glucose concentration was 400 mg per dl (22.2 mmol per L) upon arrival. When tested the following morning, fasting blood glucose was 350 mg per dl (19.5 mmol per L). He has a positive family history for type 1 diabetes mellitus.

He was admitted to the hospital for further testing, was put on insulin therapy, and met with a staff dietitian. He was discharged and told to be careful at practice, to monitor his blood glucose levels, and to be compliant with medications. On the 1st day of training camp, the team dietitian

Sample Exercise Prescription for People With Diabetes Mellitus

Warm-up typically consists of 5 to 10 minutes of low-intensity aerobic activity (typically in the activity in which you will participate, or you can walk or jog slowly). The warm-up is important because it prepares the skeletal muscles, heart, and lungs for a progressive increase in exercise intensity.

After a short warm-up, stretch the muscles for 5 to 10 minutes. Be careful not to bounce. Instead, stretch gently and slowly.

Exercise for 30 to 60 minutes, depending on the intensity. If it is easier for you to exercise in short bouts throughout the day, do so. The goal is to accumulate 30 to 60 minutes total.

The cool-down period is about 15 minutes long. Gradually bring the heart rate down to its pre-exercise level. During this period, walk slowly and then stretch slowly. Avoid standing in one place or sitting right away to prevent venous pooling in the ankles, which could cause you to pass out.

From S.L. Volpe, S.B. Sabelawski, and C.R. Mohr, 2007, *Fitness nutrition for special dietary needs* (Champaign, IL: Human Kinetics).

---

arrived in the middle of afternoon practice. K.S. staggered into the training room complaining of dizziness and feeling as if he was going to pass out. His blood glucose concentration was 60 mg per dl (3.3 mmol per L). He drank a high-carbohydrate energy drink and ate a sports bar. When he retested his blood glucose, it was 250 mg per dl (13.9 mmol per L).

I met with him to review his insulin regime, diet, and training schedule. Because he had been diagnosed with type 1 diabetes mellitus less than 2 weeks earlier, K.S. was in a state of shock and denial. He mentioned several times that there was no way he could have diabetes mellitus; after all, he was a young, healthy professional athlete. He was angry, upset, and frightened. We spent a lot of time talking about the need to take care of his health, with reassurances from the coaching and training staff that doing so would be the first priority. After he was assured that his place on the team would be secure, he was more open to discussing his diabetes management. His nutrition screening form, which all players must complete, revealed that he had good eating habits—three to four meals a day, two meals out per week, and food preferences of chicken, turkey and ham sandwiches, fruits and vegetables, and some frozen dinners. He is allergic to fish and does not eat fried foods. His typical daily fluid intake is 8 to 10 glasses per day, and he drinks more than 5 glasses during exercise.

The main concerns were the following:

- Replace lost weight
- Prevent blood glucose fluctuations
- Have a plan of action to deal with decreases in blood glucose levels
- Find palatable sugar-free options for beverages and desserts
- Work with him and his wife to develop an appropriate meal pattern

I met with K.S. to formulate a meal plan and discuss easy-to-obtain snacks to have available during practices and games. I then reviewed this information with our training staff and gave the food service staff some menu options for K.S. for grab-and-go meals after practice.

He had a few incidents that year when he forgot to take his insulin with him to an away game and was not able to play because he waited until just before the game to tell the training staff. On other occasions, he did not want to follow the eating plan before games and then experienced low blood glucose levels that required him to sit out part of the game.

After the season was over, K.S., his wife, and I met again to formulate an off-season eating plan, without the stresses of the intense training and travel during the season. He was able to implement the guidelines, bring his weight back to 319 lb (145 kg), and was willing to monitor his blood glucose concentrations several times a day without being asked. He has become involved with local support groups and is now a role model for others with diabetes mellitus.

Leslie Bonci, MPH, RD, LDN
Team Nutritionist, Pittsburgh Steelers
Pittsburgh, Pennsylvania

CHAPTER
8

Eating Disorders and Disordered Eating

CHAPTER OVERVIEW

- Types of eating disorders and disordered eating
- Identification and treatment
- Nutrition and physical activity recommendations
- Case studies

Eating disorders have become a public struggle for many professional and world-class athletes. Eating disorders and disordered eating are now in the spotlight. Both problems can be harmful and dramatically increase an athlete's risk for a variety of health issues, such as loss of bone mass, gastrointestinal problems, delayed menarche, impaired immune function, and even death. The increasing awareness of disordered eating and eating disorders has led to more effective treatments. Furthermore, greater awareness has helped families and friends become attuned to the signs and symptoms of these disorders.

This chapter touches on a variety of key concepts with regard to eating disorders and disordered eating. For detail on both topics, please refer to *Disordered Eating Among Athletes: A Comprehensive Guide for Health Professionals* by Katherine Beals (2004) and *Eating Disorders: A Clinical Guide to Counseling and Treatment* by Monika Woolsey (2002).

TYPES OF EATING DISORDERS AND DISORDERED EATING

Eating disorders and disordered eating affect a large number of women, but because the type and severity of disordered eating vary considerably,

many go undiagnosed. Disordered eating and eating disorders are serious and can lead to death if not treated. The first part of this chapter discusses the types of disordered eating and eating disorders.

Eating Disorders

Eating disorders are among the most widespread psychiatric problems affecting adolescent women today (Kreipe & Bindorf, 2000), and more than 90% of those with eating disorders are women (Office on Women's Health, 2000). Eating disorders are a worldwide problem, affecting all ethnic, socioeconomic, and cultural groups (Office on Women's Health). Eating disorders can result in morbidity and mortality if left untreated (Pritts & Sussman, 2003). Furthermore, eating disorders (and other disordered eating behaviors) are linked to other negative health behaviors such as tobacco, alcohol, and marijuana use; suicide attempts; unprotected sexual activity; and delinquency (Office on Women's Health).

An eating disorder affects approximately 1% to 4% of young women in the United States (Kreipe & Bindorf, 2000). The constant preoccupation with body weight, distorted body perception, and improper eating behaviors all lead to adverse physiological, psychological, and social consequences (Office on Women's Health, 2000). Some of the physiological changes that

The text from the heading "Types of Eating Disorders and Disordered Eating" to the heading "Female Athlete Triad" is a condensation of material from the National Institutes of Mental Health web site, www.nimh.nih.gov/publicat/eatingdisorders, and is adapted with the permission of the NIMH.

social consequences (Office on Women's Health, 2000). Some of the physiological changes that occur are an increase in body hair for warmth (lanugo), a decrease in metabolic rate, electrolyte imbalances, dehydration, cardiac problems, and osteoporosis. Psychologically, people with eating disorders experience depression, anxiety, and substance abuse. Death rates associated with eating disorders are among the highest of any mental illness amid this group (Office on Women's Health). The three most common eating disorders are ***anorexia nervosa***, ***bulimia nervosa***, and binge-eating disorder (Office on Women's Health). Females are more likely to develop one of these eating disorders than males are; approximately 5% to 15% of people with anorexia nervosa or bulimia nervosa and 35% of those with binge-eating disorder are males (Andersen, 1995; Spitzer et al., 1993).

Anorexia Nervosa

Anorexia nervosa is an eating disorder in which people starve themselves, although they are already thin (and can become dangerously thin) (National Institute of Mental Health [NIMH], 2001). Those with anorexia nervosa have an intense fear of gaining weight, and despite being severely underweight, they have a distorted body image, which is why they continue to starve themselves. Self-starvation is a form of control; people with anorexia are pleased with the fact that they are able to eat very little or nothing at all, especially in public.

Symptoms of anorexia nervosa include refusal to eat; opposition to sustaining a body weight at or above normal body weight for age and height; intense fear of gaining weight or becoming fat, despite being severely underweight; distorted body image; denial of the extremely low body weight; unwarranted influence of body weight on self-evaluation; and, in females who have reached puberty, oligomenorrhea (infrequent menstrual cycles, usually less than six per year) or amenorrhea (lack of menstruation) (NIMH, 2001). People with anorexia nervosa are usually perfectionists and overachievers, and although they may appear to be in control, they typically experience low self-worth and low self-confidence, and place undue criticism upon themselves. Often, they are concerned about pleasing others (Office on Women's Health, 2000).

Individuals with anorexia nervosa starve themselves in a number of ways. These prac-

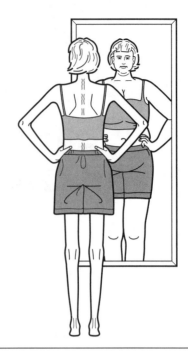

Figure 8.1 People with anorexia nervosa are incapable of seeing themselves as they really are. No matter how thin they become, they falsely see themselves as fat.

Reprinted, by permission, from S.J. Shultz, P. Houglum, and D. Perrin, 2005, *Examination of musculoskeletal injuries*, 2nd ed. (Champaign, IL: Human Kinetics), 615.

tices include refusing to eat (often by moving food around on a plate at meals but not eating the meal); self-induced vomiting; overexercising; using laxatives, diuretics, or enemas; extreme dieting; and fasting (Office on Women's Health, 2000).

A number of factors may cause anorexia nervosa, such as a comment from a coach to an athlete that losing a little weight would be helpful. Typically, however, anorexia nervosa begins after a traumatic event in a person's life (for example, during puberty or when one leaves home for the first time) (Office on Women's Health, 2000). Regardless of the cause, this serious illness needs to be addressed quickly to prevent major adverse outcomes. But because people with anorexia nervosa often dress with layers, their weight loss may not be noticeable for some time, even by family members. Therefore, friends and family members must be alert for signs of this illness, such as eating little, overexercising, obsessing about food, and so on.

Because people with anorexia nervosa are starving themselves, the signs of starvation will be visible. These indicators include severe thinness, brittle hair and nails, dry skin, lanugo,

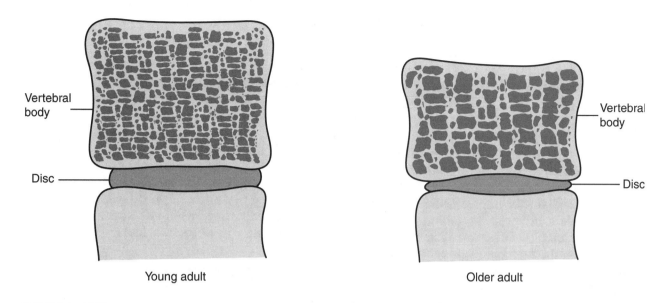

Vertebral body

Disc

Young adult

Vertebral body

Disc

Older adult

Figure 8.2   Notice the dense lattice of bony tissue in the normal vertebra on the left versus the age-related osteoporotic loss of the bony network in the vertebra on the right. A similarly severe bone loss can occur in young people who have developed osteoporosis as a side effect of long-term anorexia nervosa.

Reprinted, by permission, from B. Abernethy et al., 2004, *The biophysical foundations of human movement,* 2nd ed. (Champaign, IL: Human Kinetics), 46.

decreased metabolic rate, decreased heart rate, inability to tolerate cold, anemia, decreased muscle mass, decreased fat mass, amenorrhea or oligomenorrhea, constipation and occasional diarrhea, and joint inflammation (Office on Women's Health, 2000). Long-term consequences of anorexia nervosa include dysrhythmias (irregular heartbeat), osteoporosis, clinical depression, substance abuse, personality disorders, and increased risk of suicide (Office on Women's Health). About 1 in 10 women who have anorexia nervosa will die of starvation, cardiac arrest, or other medical complication resulting from the disorder (NIMH, 2001).

Bulimia Nervosa

Bulimia nervosa is characterized by secretive binge eating of abnormal amounts of foods followed by some type of purging. The purging is usually self-induced vomiting, but it can also occur through abuse of laxatives, diet pills, diuretics, excessive exercise ("exercise bulimia"), or bouts of fasting (Office on Women's Health, 2000). Purging can range from twice a week to more than twice a day, and the person may purge through a combination of methods. Approximately 1.1% to 4.2% of women have bulimia nervosa during their lifetime (American Psychiatric Association, 2000). Because people with bulimia nervosa binge

and purge in private, and because they do absorb many of the nutrients and much of the energy that they consume, their body weight is typically within or above the normal range for their height and age. Therefore, people can hide this disorder from others for years. Nonetheless, individuals with bulimia nervosa fear gaining weight, always desire to lose weight, and are not satisfied with their bodies (NIMH, 2001).

Persons with bulimia nervosa typically have a difficult time controlling their impulses, and dealing with pressure. Although bulimia nervosa occurs separately from anorexia nervosa, about half of those with anorexia nervosa develop bulimia nervosa (Office on Women's Health, 2000).

A number of complications also result from bulimia nervosa, including electrolyte imbalances because of purging. These imbalances can damage cardiac muscle, possibly leading to cardiac arrest (which can also result from an imbalance in potassium because of purging— through either self-induced vomiting, laxative abuse, or diuretic abuse) (Office on Women's Health, 2000; Horton, 1988). Self-induced vomiting can also lead to esophageal inflammation, erosion of tooth enamel, and damage to the salivary glands (Office on Women's Health). Tooth erosion and cracked gums and lips may be signs to look for if bulimia nervosa is suspected. Those with bulimia nervosa often have drug or alcohol addiction and may practice compulsive stealing (Office on Women's Health). In addition, they typically suffer from clinical depression, anxiety, and obsessive-compulsive disorder (OCD) (Office on Women's Health).

Binge-Eating Disorder

Binge-eating disorder, one of the newest clinically observed eating disorders, is characterized by repeated bouts of uncontrolled eating. But in binge-eating disorder, unlike bulimia nervosa, the person does not purge and thus may become obese (NIMH, 2001; Office on Women's Health, 2000). Estimates are that from 2% to 5% of the population in the United States has suffered from binge-eating disorder within a 6-month period (Bruce & Agras, 1992; Spitzer et al., 1993). Binge-eating disorder usually occurs in late adolescence or in the early 20s, and it may occur after a person has lost a large amount of weight after being on a low-energy diet. The prevalence of binge-eating disorder may be quite high in people who are participating in weight-control programs (Office on Women's Health, 2000).

Some symptoms of binge-eating disorder include consuming a large amount of food within a distinct period accompanied by a sense of a lack of control; eating much more quickly than normal; eating beyond satiation; consuming large amounts of food without the feeling of hunger; eating alone; feeling disgusted, depressed, or guilty after a binge-eating episode; and engaging in binge eating about 2 days per week for at least 6 months (NIMH, 2001).

People with binge-eating disorder do not practice purging as do those with anorexia nervosa and bulimia nervosa. Therefore, people with binge-eating disorder are typically overweight or obese because of their high energy intake. Furthermore, the feelings of disgust, embarrassment, and shame can lead to another bingeing episode, thus creating a vicious cycle (NIMH, 2001).

The medical complications associated with binge-eating disorder are the same as those observed with obesity: increased risk of type 2 diabetes mellitus, heart disease, hypertension, certain cancers, and osteoarthritis, to name a few. In addition, people with binge-eating disorder often suffer from depression (Office on Women's Health, 2000).

Eating Disorders Not Otherwise Specified

Eating disorders not otherwise specified, often referred to as EDNOS, is a classification of eating disorders that does not meet any standards of the previously mentioned eating disorders (Office on Women's Health, 2000). For example, a person with EDNOS may practice some behaviors of bulimia nervosa but may not practice purging as often as has been clinically defined for that disorder. Thus, a person with EDNOS regularly practices disordered eating but not so specifically that it can be placed into one particular category.

Disordered Eating

Disordered eating refers to complicated eating behaviors, such as restraining food consumption, bingeing, or purging (by vomiting, use of diuretics or laxatives, or overexercising), that occur less habitually or are less severe than those necessary to meet the full criteria for the diagnosis of an eating disorder. Disordered eating can result from an illness, wanting to change one's appearance, a traumatic occurrence, or to prepare for an athletic event (Office on Women's Health, 2000). Although disordered eating does not always lead to a full-blown eating disorder, people who display such eating behaviors should be monitored to prevent an eating disorder from occurring.

Female Athlete Triad

The female athlete triad is characterized as the combination of disordered eating (including all levels of unhealthy eating behaviors), amenorrhea (the absence of menstruation), and osteoporosis (porous bones; more than 2.5 standard deviations below average for young adults) (Hobart & Smucker, 2000; Otis, Drinkwater, Johnson, Loucks, & Wilmore, 1997). The female athlete triad was first established in 1992 at a consensus conference hosted by the Task Force on Women's Issues of the American College of Sports Medicine (Otis et al., 1997; Yeager, Agostini, Nattiv, & Drinkwater, 1993). In 1997 the American College of Sports Medicine published a position stand on the female athlete triad (Otis et al., 1997).

The position of the American College of Sports Medicine on the female athlete triad is paraphrased as follows (Otis et al., 1997):

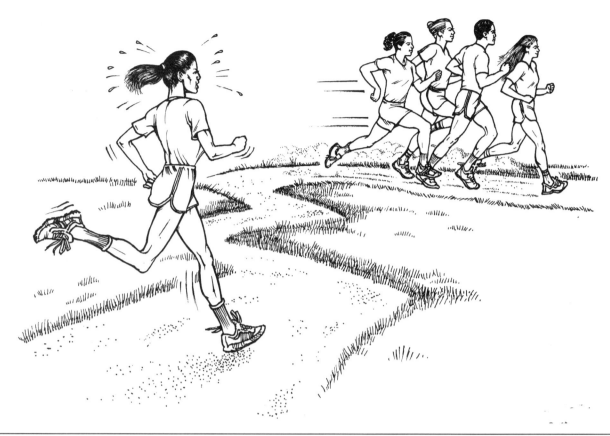

Figure 8.3 If women with the female athletic triad can face the fact that their disorder is causing them to perform more poorly than their healthier peers, they may be motivated to deal realistically with their condition.

Reprinted, by permission, from N. Clark, 1996, *Nancy Clark's sports nutrition guidebook,* 2nd ed. (Champaign, IL: Human Kinetics), 273.

- The female athlete triad is a serious condition that can affect all girls and women, not only elite athletes but also girls and women who participate in a spectrum of physical activity levels.

- These disorders are usually triggered by internal and external pressures for girls and women to achieve an unrealistically low body weight.

- Because the female athlete triad is often denied and underreported, health professionals, especially those working in the area of sports, must be made aware of the signs and symptoms of the female athlete triad.

- Girls or women with one component of the female athlete triad should be screened for the other two components. Preparticipation exams offer the easiest way to conduct the screening.

- All levels of people who work with girls and women in sports should recognize the signs and symptoms of the female athlete triad, and they should not place undue pressure on girls and women to achieve below-normal body weight. They should be trained to know how to speak to their female athletes in ways that will not result in disordered eating, which can lead to the other facets of the female athlete triad.

- Parents should learn about the warning signs of the female athlete triad so that they do not pressure their daughters to lose weight.

- Sports governing bodies need to educate coaches and all athletic personnel about the signs and symptoms of the female athlete triad. Coaches and other personnel must understand how to conduct themselves among female athletes so that they do not place undue pressures on them, either inadvertently or directly. A mechanism should be in place to monitor coaches as well.

- Physically active girls and women need to be educated about nutrition, healthy eating, and the signs of the female athlete triad. They should be immediately referred to a medical professional if they possess one component of the female athlete triad.
- More research is required to assess the prevalence, causes, and treatment of the female athlete triad.

IDENTIFICATION AND TREATMENT

Estimates of the prevalence of disordered eating and eating disorders among athletes vary widely because of the different definitions applied to disordered eating and eating disorders, varied screening tools and assessment tools used, and different populations studied. Estimates range from 1% to 62% in female athletes and 0% to 57% in male athletes (Andersen, 1992; Byrne & McLean, 2001). Therefore, health professionals must learn to identify signs and symptoms of eating disorders and disordered eating, warning signs, and other tools used to assess these conditions.

Identifying Eating Disorders and Disordered Eating

Many people are able to conceal their eating disorders, especially those with bulimia nervosa, because they are often of normal body weight or slightly overweight. Thus, identifying someone who has an eating disorder may be difficult. We have previously discussed many signs and symptoms. The United States Department of Health and Human Services has put together a list of warning signs for family members and friends to be aware of should they suspect an eating disorder. See the section *"Warning Signs of Eating Disorders."*

Clients with eating disorders or disordered eating often deny that they have a problem and try to hide their behaviors or minimize the severity of their disorder. Those with eating disorders or disordered eating are often concerned that others will learn of their condition. They are usually embarrassed by their own behavior, and they may feel that their parents and coaches will disapprove, shame them, and ultimately withhold them

---

Warning Signs of Eating Disorders

A person with anorexia may

- eat only "safe" foods, usually those low in energy and fat;
- have odd rituals, such as cutting food into small pieces;
- spend more time playing with food than eating it;
- cook meals for others without eating;
- engage in compulsive exercising;
- dress in layers to hide weight loss; or
- spend less time with family and friends, and become more isolated, withdrawn, and secretive.

A person with bulimia may

- become secretive about food and spend a lot of time thinking about and planning the next binge;
- take repeated trips to the bathroom, particularly after eating;
- steal food or hoard it in strange places; or
- engage in compulsive exercising.

A person who displays any of these behaviors should be taken to a physician, nutritionist, or other professional with expertise in diagnosing eating disorders.

Adapted from NIH Publication No. 01-4901, 2001, courtesy of the National Institute of Mental Health.

---

from athletic participation. You must therefore be sensitive to the situation, but firm, of course. You must be a good listener as you approach the athlete whom you suspect of having a problem with disordered eating or eating disorders. If you are working with a female athlete who has become convinced of your empathy and desire to help, you can gently begin to inquire about the issues listed on *"Screening History for the Female Athlete Triad"* (page 135). If you approach the athlete in a timely fashion, demonstrate sincere concern for her well-being and give her some time to admit to her condition. She may trust you enough to be straightforward with you. Although treating this condition early is the best way to preserve the

Screening History for the Female Athlete Triad

The following information should be obtained when screening for the female athlete triad:

Menstrual history

- Age at menarche
- Frequency and duration of menstrual cycles
- Longest time without menstruation
- Last menstrual period
- Physical signs of ovulation, such as cervical mucus change or menstrual cramps
- Hormonal therapy taken previously and currently

Diet history

- Food consumption in the past 24 hours
- List of any forbidden foods
- Highest and lowest body weight since menarche

- Happiness with current body weight
- Ideal body weight according to the patient
- Disordered eating practices: bingeing and purging
- Use of laxatives, diuretics, or diet pills

Exercise history

- Exercise frequency, training, and intensity for the sport (hours per day, days per week)
- Additional exercise outside required training
- History of previous fractures
- History of overuse injuries

From S.L. Volpe, S.B. Sabelawski, and C.R. Mohr, 2007, *Fitness nutrition for special dietary needs* (Champaign, IL: Human Kinetics). Reprinted, by permission, from J.A. Hobart and D.R. Smucker, 2000, "The female athlete triad," *American Family Physician* 61(11): 3357-3364.

---

athlete's health, patience is needed. The athlete may ignore a heavy-handed approach.

Treatment of Eating Disorders

Treatment of eating disorders requires a team approach. At a minimum, the team should include a physician, a psychologist or psychiatrist, a registered dietitian who specializes in eating disorders, and an exercise physiologist. Sometimes a social worker is necessary, especially if the home environment is the major root of the problem. The earlier the problem is diagnosed, the better the chance of recovery and the lower the risk that other medical conditions will occur or persist (for example, heart problems or osteoporosis). For additional resources on eating disorders and disordered eating, see *"Resources for Eating Disorders and Disordered Eating"* (page 136).

General Principles of Treatment

If the person has had the eating disorder for a long time and has become so thin that the disorder is life threatening, he or she must be hospitalized. Typically, tube feeding or total parenteral nutrition (TPN) is required. The person may fight this intervention at first, but this is a life-or-death issue. Increased energy intake, even through tube feeding and TPN, needs to be gradual to avoid straining the internal organs, especially the heart and kidneys.

After a person has become stable, the next step is to increase energy intake to more normal levels so that weight gain occurs. But the crucial aspect here is to teach the person how to eat properly so that he or she does not become overweight. The person will then be more likely to eat normally again.

Exercise should also be part of the treatment equation. Although the person may have used exercise, like food, in an unhealthy way, it needs to be added in a positive, gradual manner, just as food was incorporated. Becoming comfortable with exercising with others and learning to enjoy exercise will take time, but it can be done. Focusing on exercises that the person enjoys is a useful approach, but he or she must be taught to exercise sensibly, not senselessly.

Weight-Gain Recommendations

Although every person will have different weight-gain goals, these general guidelines for weight gain are suitable for people with eating disorders:

Resources for Eating Disorders and Disordered Eating

Several resources listed here can be helpful for people with eating disorders and their families. The Office on Women's Health (United States Department of Health and Human Services) sponsors BodyWise, an educational program targeted to middle school children to decrease the prevalence of eating disorders (www. womenshealth.gov). The Office on Women's Health also sponsors the National Women's Health Information Center, which provides information on women's health, including eating disorders. In addition, the Office on Women's Health supports an educational program called Girl Power! that offers positive messages and accurate health information to young girls ages 9 to 13 (www.health.org/gpower/).

The Food and Drug Administration (FDA) has a Web site that provides information on diet and nutrition to women and adolescents (www.fda.gov/womens/informat.html). *FDA Consumer* magazine occasionally prints articles with vital health information for teenagers, called Teen Scene articles, which are accessible electronically at www.fda.gov/oc/opacom/kids/html/7teens.htm.

Office on Women's Health
200 Independence Avenue SW
Room 712E
Washington, DC 20201
202-690-7650
www.womenshealth.gov

Food and Drug Administration
5600 Fishers Lane
Rockville, MD 20857
888-INFO-FDA
www.fda.gov.

National Institute of Mental Health Public
    Inquiries Section
6001 Executive Boulevard, Room 8184, MSC
    9663
Bethesda, MD 20892
301-443-4513
http://www.nimh.nih.gov.

Weight-Control Information Network (WIN)
(Sponsored by the National Institute of Diabetes and Diseases of the Kidney)
1 WIN WAY
Bethesda, MD 20892-3665
202-828-1025
http://win.niddk.nih.gov/index.htm

National Eating Disorders Association
603 Stewart Street, Suite 803
Seattle, WA 98101
800-931-2237
www.nationaleatingdisorders.org

National Association of Anorexia Nervosa and
    Associated Disorders
Box 7
Highland Park, IL 60035
847-831-3438
www.anad.org

Pennsylvania Educational Network on Eating
    Disorders
7805 McKnight Road
Pittsburgh, PA 15237
412-366-9966
www.pened.org

American Family Physician patient handout with information on the female athlete triad: www.aafp. org/afp/20000601/3367ph.html

From S.L. Volpe, S.B. Sabelawski, and C.R. Mohr, 2007, *Fitness nutrition for special dietary needs* (Champaign, IL: Human Kinetics). Provided by the Office on Women's Health (2000), courtesy of the U.S. Department of Health and Human Services.

- Slow, gradual weight gain to minimize stress on the heart and kidneys
- Weight gain of no more than 0.5 to 1 lb per week (0.23 to 0.45 kg per week), achieved by slowly increasing energy intake
- Initial increase of about 1,400 kcal per week (5,852 kJ per week), achieved by adding about 200 kcal per day (836 kJ per day) and resulting in a 0.5 lb per week (0.23 kg per week) weight gain
- Eventual goal of increasing energy intake by 500 kcal per day (2,090 kJ per day), leading to a 1.0 lb per week (0.45 kg per week) weight gain until normal weight is attained
- Stabilization of patient's energy intake to maintain normal weight

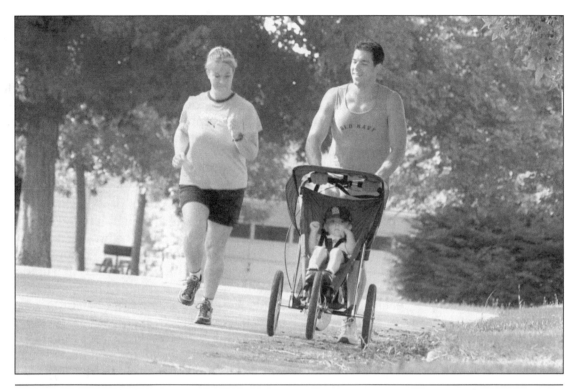

This couple has found an enjoyable and social form of exercise that fits their lifestyle. Such experiences are usually foreign to people with eating disorders. Part of your job is to help those people identify normal and healthy forms of exercise they can enjoy with other people.

Although weight gain is the major concern (or weight loss, in the case of binge-eating disorder; see information on weight loss in chapter 6), maintaining muscle mass is also a concern, for both the health and the psychological well-being of the person. Maintaining muscle mass will also help prevent the person from becoming overweight. Therefore, after the person becomes stable, incorporating healthy exercise and physical activity into his or her life is important. Again, the process should be gradual. Even if the person had been training for a marathon before treatment, exercise needs to be incorporated slowly for health concerns (to reduce strain on the heart) and to allow the person to accept exercise as a healthy, fun part of life, not as something that is mandatory to burn kilocalories.

NUTRITION AND PHYSICAL ACTIVITY RECOMMENDATIONS

Nutrition also plays an important role in the treatment of people with eating disorders or disordered eating. A team of health profession-als that includes a psychiatrist or psychologist, an internal medicine physician, a registered dietitian, and perhaps a social worker should be working with the patient. Psychological treatment should be the cornerstone, but nutrition counseling by a registered dietitian who specializes in treating eating disorders and disordered eating is crucial.

Nutrition

A person with an eating disorder has relatively high nutrient needs. The person needs not only more overall energy but also a good balance of micronutrients to help with repair. For example, zinc, iron, calcium, vitamin C, and vitamin D will all be important nutrients for healing. Nonetheless, a well-balanced diet that includes all nutrients will be required. Because the individual's energy intake will be gradually increased, a multivitamin and mineral supplement is typically prescribed to provide the much-needed micronutrients. Over time, after dietary intake has become well balanced, supplementation may be discontinued. But if the person still has problems with osteoporosis, for example (which is likely because even in recovery, bone density will not return to what it was before the eating disorder developed), he or she may require increased calcium intake. Similarly, the person may need greater iron intake if he or she remains anemic. But returning to a more normal diet as soon as possible is important so that eating habits become less of a focus to the patient.

All members of the health care team need to communicate with one another to facilitate the patient's recovery. Although the condition is primarily a psychological issue, the registered dietitian plays a vital role in the total treatment and must be kept abreast of the progress of the patient from a psychological standpoint. In fact, all members of the team should provide information to the others with regard to how the patient is progressing in each aspect of recovery. The ultimate goal is to identify the underlying psychological issues involved in the development of the eating disorder or disordered eating and then to normalize behaviors and body weight. After becoming aware of the mental and emotional aspects of the patient, the

registered dietitian can focus on making positive changes in the patient's eating behaviors to address specific energy and nutrient concerns, deficiencies, and so forth. Nutrient deficiencies can range from moderate to severe, so addressing these concerns initially is crucial, likely through supplementation because the patient will be resistant to dramatic changes in food intake. In conjunction with the primary care physician on the team, the registered dietitian should address these concerns immediately to prevent problems from progressing.

The sample meal plan that follows is an example of a meal that could be provided to an athlete who has an eating disorder or disordered eating. As always, you must work with each unique situation and client to monitor progress and make changes as necessary. Although this meal plan is still relatively low in energy because it is designed for the early stages of recovery from disordered eating or an eating disorder, it provides an array of foods and nutrients, colorful fruits and vegetables, and whole grains to ensure the inclusion of the required nutrients.

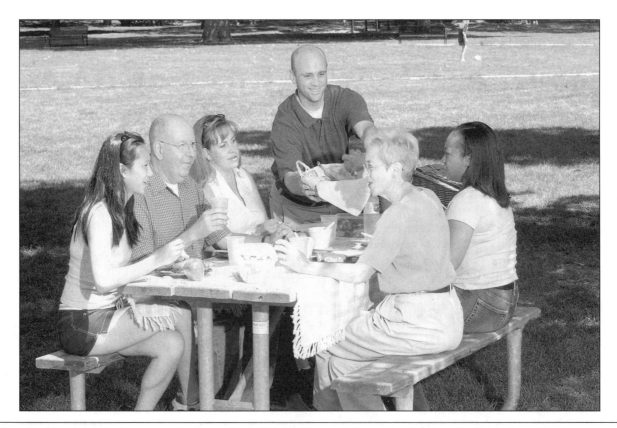

You should emphasize to your patients or clients the positive social aspects of eating. Facing and wanting to overcome the isolation that often comes with disordered eating or eating disorders can be a powerful motivator for them to take action toward healing.

Sample Meal Plan for People With Eating Disorders and Disordered Eating

This meal plan provides a gradual increase in energy intake for a person early in recovery from an eating disorder. The plan supplies a healthy variety of nutrients, food choices, vitamins, and minerals. As with the plans in other chapters, this meal plan is only a guideline. Each client should be treated individually. Thus, this meal plan can be altered based on the severity of the eating disorder or disordered eating, gender, level of training, likes, dislikes, allergies, and so on.

Breakfast

- 1/2 cup of Grape Nuts Flakes cereal = 113 g
- 1/2 cup of skim milk = 120 ml
- 1/4 cup of strawberries = 57 g
- 1/2 cup of orange juice = 120 ml

Snack

- 1 apple = 80 g
- 8 oz of water = 240 ml

Lunch

- Turkey sandwich
    - 1 oz of unprocessed sliced turkey breast = 28 g
    - 1 slice of whole-wheat bread = 40 g
    - 1 slice each of lettuce and tomato = 30 g
    - 1 tsp of mustard = 5 g
- 1 cup of skim milk = 240 ml

Snack

- 1/4 cup of low-fat cottage cheese = 60 g
- 8 oz of water = 240 ml

Dinner

- 2 oz of baked salmon = 60 g
- 1/2 cup of brown rice = 60 g
- 1/2 cup of steamed broccoli = 56 g
- 8 oz of water = 240 ml

Snack

- 8 oz of low-fat vanilla yogurt = 227 g
- 4 oz of water = 120 ml

This sample meal plan provides at least 100% of the Dietary Reference Intakes (DRI) for energy, protein, fiber, vitamins A, C, E, B_6, B_{12}, thiamin, riboflavin, niacin, folate, calcium, iron, magnesium, phosphorus, zinc, and approximately

- 1,500 kcal (6,270 kJ),
- 65 g of protein,
- 50 g of fat,
- 17 g of fiber, and
- 2,000 mg of sodium.

From S.L. Volpe, S.B. Sabelawski, and C.R. Mohr, 2007, *Fitness nutrition for special dietary needs* (Champaign, IL: Human Kinetics).

Nutritionally, the first concern is to address any deficiencies. Because the person is either restricting energy or purging, he or she is at a high risk for nutrient deficiencies. Therefore, besides providing supplementation, you should work with the client or patient to provide the greatest variety of foods possible. Although initially the amount of each food will be small, providing variety will increase the likelihood that the individual will include it later in his or her regular intake.

Besides correcting deficiencies, the registered dietitian must also manage the person's body weight by encouraging an increase in energy intake. People afflicted with eating disorders or disordered eating will resist an immediate increase in energy intake. A small but gradual

increase in energy will increase adherence. Adding basic high-nutrient foods, such as yogurt, fruits, and skim milk, is a good place to begin. These foods are high in micronutrients that are often lacking in those with eating disorders or disordered eating. As recovery progresses, the variety of foods can be increased. The goal should be to correct nutritional deficiencies and stabilize body weight. When the patient or client has reached that goal, the dietitian can recommend small increases in energy to match the needs of the client.

As the person's recovery progresses, the portions of each of the foods can be increased. The key is for each meal to include some fruits or vegetables for their nutrient quality, some whole grains for their unique nutrients and fiber, and some lean protein to maintain or help build muscle mass as energy needs increase.

Exercise

Here are some general principles that you should incorporate into your usual exercise prescription strategies:

• Because of the negative connotation that exercise has had in those with eating disorders or disordered eating, such clients should be progressed gradually to higher levels of exercise. They should be taught to enjoy exercise and physical activity, to focus not on the energy being burned but on the muscle mass that will be preserved and the health benefits that they will gain. Thus, you must work with each client to determine what exercises he or she enjoys. Activities such as walking, bike riding, or swimming may be activities that some athletes do not consider exercise, yet they provide important health benefits. Encourage the client to perform other daily activities, such as walking with the dog or with friends, gardening, dancing, and so forth. These activities expend some energy, but they are not competitive pursuits that could compel the person to work out at greater intensity and hence revert to using exercise as a type of purging.

• Encourage your client to use behavioral strategies to adopt enjoyable levels of exercise and physical activity. For example, writing in a journal about mental and physical feelings can help a person with disordered eating or an eating disorder overcome some of the psychological pain associated with this struggle. Health professionals should not use anthropometric measurements because the process encourages preoccupation with the body. The last thing that the person with disordered eating or an eating disorder needs is any sort of motivation to strive for the perfect body. Another important aspect of recovery is providing a comfortable, inviting atmosphere where people can talk openly about body image, healthful eating practices, and weight management. Again, the team approach is critical to recovery.

• Aerobic and resistance training should be incorporated and increased gradually over time. Healthy doses of aerobic exercise must be clearly distinguished from anorexia athletica, a condition in which exercise becomes excessive. Aerobic exercise is crucial for overall health, particularly for strengthening the cardiovascular system, but the amount needs to be monitored to ensure it is within normal, recommended amounts to remain healthy. Resistance training is important for maintaining muscle mass, gaining weight, and strengthening potentially weakened bones. Providing information about how strengthened muscles can improve performance may help those with disordered eating or eating disorders understand the benefits of training, because many will not want to accept the weight gain that may result from increased lean muscle mass that may result from weight training. To increase adherence, the person should begin weight training with a resistance that is comfortable but challenging. The intensity and activity should be increased on an individual basis. For optimal performance, energy intake should likewise increase. Depending on the severity of the eating disorder or disordered eating, these sessions may have to be monitored so that the person remains safe throughout the training session.

• The person with the eating disorder or disordered eating must understand that some weight gain will occur but that a healthy amount of exercise balanced with healthy eating will result in a weight gain that will be primarily muscle.

Myths About Weight Gain in Recovery From Eating Disorders and Disordered Eating

Eating disorders and disordered eating, as you have learned in this chapter, are multifaceted disorders that require a team approach for a healthy recovery. One of the biggest fears of a person with an eating disorder or disordered eating is that any weight gain will be as fat. This is a myth. With proper consumption of healthy meals, a gradual increase in energy intake that provides a good balance of macronutrients and micronutrients, and a healthy exercise program, the weight gain will be primarily in the form of muscle. Granted, the person will gain some fat, but a person with anorexia nervosa must regain some fat for normal physiological functioning.

• The number of minutes or repetitions of workouts needs to be downplayed somewhat. Exercise and eating were all negative in the past, so for recovery, the behavioral strategies mentioned earlier in this chapter need to be used to encourage a good lifestyle balance of exercise and eating.

CASE STUDIES

Our guest dietitians and nutritionists have provided us with four case studies in this chapter. Three involve women, and one is about a man. All have eating disorders. You will see recurrent themes in these poignant case studies: Weight gain was difficult for all clients to achieve, weight gain was gradual, and exercise was part of the process for each.

Female Dancer With Anorexia Nervosa

C.V. is a 17-year-old dance student who presented at 94 lb (42.7 kg) and 63.25 in. (160.7 cm). She had amenorrhea. The last time the dancer had menstruated was 1 1/2 years ago at 100 lb (45.5 kg). She had no history of stress fractures. She had seen a physician experienced in the female athlete triad and the demands of dance. The physician suggested a weight of 98 to 100 lb (44.5 to 45.5 kg) as a more appropriate weight, a weight at which C.V. might begin menstruation. She was to be reassessed again. C.V. was taking a One-A-Day multivitamin and mineral supplement.

This dancer had seen another nutritionist who recommended a program that eliminated all refined foods, lowered fat intake dramatically, and was low in total energy. The dancer was extremely motivated to eat healthy and was compliant with the program, but she went too far. Review of her food journal showed that the dancer prepared and ate foods like curried quinoa with lentils and spinach, included steamed fish in her diet, and ate a handful of nuts. Although she was consuming healthy foods, her total energy intake was insufficient. She did not consume red meat.

C.V. misunderstood the role of saturated fat. We reviewed the components of the female athlete triad, the need for fat and protein in her diet, the body-fat level required for normal physiological functioning, and her overall energy needs. She was extremely receptive to all that I presented to her, except for the need to include fat in her diet. Because of this, I suggested that she start by consuming 20 g of fat per day. She began by adding low-fat dairy products but then excluded other foods. We slowly increased her fat intake. She gained 4 lb (1.8 kg) to reach 98 lb (44.5 kg) but then lost 1.5 lb (0.68 kg) to fall back to 96.5 lb (43.9 kg). Following this slight setback, she agreed to consume filet mignon and eggs once or twice per week. She also agreed to switch to 1% milk (instead of consuming only soy milk). She decreased her intake of nuts. We brainstormed about snacks that she liked and felt comfortable consuming (for example, an apple with string cheese, rice cakes and hummus). She agreed to add snacks strategically around dance classes and meals. She also agreed to stop writing in her food journal to reduce her focus on food and the amounts that she consumed. She increased her body weight to 103 lb but then lost 2 lb to 101 lb (45.9 kg).

She continued to see her physician. Her blood hormone levels and body weight were still below normal. Her physician prescribed progesterone, and she resumed menstruation for one cycle. I was concerned about her tendency to overtrain. Besides going to dance classes, she worked out to become even more conditioned. We discussed the implications of overtraining versus the healthiness of conditioning. I encouraged her to speak with her physical therapist and strength and conditioning coach to determine the quantity of exercise that would promote health and conditioning but avoid the risk of overtraining.

We reviewed breakfast, lunch, and snack ideas and will do so again as the journey continues.

Heidi Skolnik MS, CDN, FACSM
Nutrition Conditioning, Inc.
Englewood Cliffs, New Jersey

Female Gymnast With Disordered Eating

Katie was a 17-year old, 5 ft 2 in. (157.5 cm), 136 lb (61.8 kg) competitive gymnast about to graduate from high school and attend a Division I university on a gymnastics scholarship. During high school, she excelled in her sport, winning several consecutive state championships in the uneven bars, balance beam, and floor exercise while maintaining a high grade point average. Given her competitive history and sport-specific scholarship, Katie expressed feeling a lot of pressure entering her 1st year of college, and she wanted to gain a competitive edge. She struggled with poor body image and believed that losing weight would not only make her a better competitor but also make her coaches like her more. Present and previous coaches had instructed Katie to lose weight, and her future coach suggested that she lose weight before arriving on campus to secure her spot on the team, which she felt she could lose at any time if she did not prove herself.

Due to the body-conscious nature of gymnastics, the prodding and disapproval from her coaches, and the pressure to maintain her scholarship at an out-of-state university, Katie believed that she was too heavy, felt fat, and wanted to lose weight. Believing that she should compete at 112 lb (50.9 kg), Katie's weight-loss goal was 24 lb (10.9 kg). Katie had recently seen a physician because of feelings of fatigue; the physician tested her for Sjogren's syndrome, which runs in her family. Sjogren's syndrome is a disorder of the immune system, with typical symptoms of xeropthalmia (dry eyes) and a dry mouth (www.mayoclinic.com/health/sjogrens-syndrome/DS00147).

Her physician also suggested the possibility that Katie had lupus (an autoimmune disease). Besides feeling fatigued, Katie had only two menstrual cycles per year and had low bone mineral density.

Although Katie had never had a sophisticated body composition test, such as underwater weighing or dual-energy X-ray absorptiometry (DEXA), visual assessment suggested that Katie was a highly fit, muscular young woman with body fat well within the expected range of a competitive athlete. Food record analysis indicated that Katie consumed about 900 kcal per day (3,762 kJ per day). Although she chose healthy foods, she was an extremely regimented, restrictive eater. At the same time, she maintained an intense training protocol, which included waking up at 5:00 a.m. to perform an hour of aerobic training (on an elliptical trainer, stair-stepper, or treadmill) before school and practicing daily after school for 3 to 4 hours.

During our first meeting, Katie, her mother, and I discussed the demands of her sport, her food preferences, weight goals, and competitive goals. Given her frame, the demands of her sport, the lack of regular menses, and her feelings of fatigue, we jointly set a more modest initial weight-loss goal of 10 to 12 lb (4.5 to 5.5 kg) and developed a calcium-rich meal plan that included pre- and postexercise snacks to provide energy

and replenish glycogen stores and lost nutrients. Katie was reluctant to increase her energy intake, although the meal plan was designed to meet her energy needs more adequately. Only "Katie-approved-foods" were included in her meal plan, which she followed with a high-degree of compliance according to food records and objective reports by her family, who were involved in her care. Katie was most successful with her pre- and postexercise snacks, which she consumed around practice, but not before her morning workout. After graduating from high school, Katie shifted her priorities to getting more sleep, modifying her morning routine, and maintaining a daily practice schedule at her gymnastics club. She took Sundays off from working out and began to eat more meals with her family.

Before her departure for college, Katie's body weight changed very little with only minor fluctuations. Nonetheless, her energy level increased, which paralleled her increased energy intake, although her reported intake was still below the level recommended to meet her training needs. Her physician ruled out both lupus and Sjogren's syndrome, although she required follow-up appointments to monitor her bone mineral density.

Katie, currently a sophomore in college, is still competing in gymnastics and maintaining a high grade point average. Her current body weight and eating habits are unknown.

Anne-Marie Nocton, MS, MPH, RD, LDN
Nutrition Consultant and Private Practice Dietitian
Knoxville, Tennessee

Male With Anorexia Nervosa and Bulimia Nervosa

Russell came to me as a referral when he was a 3rd-year student at the private college where I was practicing. He was concerned about his ability to remain in college because he had a low grade point average. He told me that he had experienced dietary problems for most of his life and that he felt that completing his education at this college was his last chance at normality. He was extremely fatigued, and his ability to concentrate was failing him. He was abnormally thin, weighing just 149 lb (67.7 kg) at 6 ft 1 in. (185.4 cm) tall. His hair was falling out, and he had a severe dry skin condition.

He came from a wealthy family, but his parents had been killed years before in a car accident.

So from an early age, Russell spent his childhood with his grandmother. She had continually abused him, constantly telling him that he was worthless, ugly, and fat. She indulged in behavior that depleted Russell's self-esteem. By the age of 13, the abuse had worn Russell out, and his body began to shut down. At a low body weight, he started college in an attempt to put distance between himself and his family. By the end of the first semester, he felt increasingly hopeless and different from other students. The situation continued to worsen.

When he was 20 years old, his physician referred him to a psychiatrist, who simply said, "Go home and eat." But he was unable to do that because he felt controlled by his internal dialogue, which told him how bad he was every time he ate. Unable to force himself to eat, except for the odd occasions, he would be compelled to binge. He eventually became extremely weak and collapsed in class one day. He was admitted into the hospital, where he was diagnosed with anorexia nervosa. His college allowed him to return to classes but strongly recommended that he see a therapist. He began seeing a psychologist from within the college once a week. She thought that his eating disorder was not as serious as diagnosed. Russell agreed with her, because as he would later admit, this finding was convenient because it masked the shame that he felt at being labeled as having anorexia nervosa, especially as a male.

Russell was obsessed with food and went to extreme measures to avoid eating. He made elaborate plans to dispose of food without anyone's knowledge, and he began exercising and taking laxatives several times a day. He continued to work with the psychologist for a year, yet his anorexia nervosa worsened. Within 15 months, following another collapse on campus, his college advised him that they could not continue to accept liability for him and that he should leave and seek treatment. This occurrence drove Russell further into a crisis. He began binge eating and taking even more laxatives to counteract any potential weight gain.

He enrolled in another college and managed to interact enough to make new friends. One of those friends, Brad, recognized some of the characteristics of anorexia nervosa from previous experience with a close family member.

Through months of gentle perseverance, Brad gradually persuaded Russell that he should not be ashamed to talk about his issue and that his situation was not unique. Russell agreed to see a nutritionist and was referred to me. We spent a lot of time talking about his feelings toward food. He iterated that he was a "master at controlling his own hunger." When asked to expand on this, Russell explained somewhat proudly that he welcomed the feeling of hunger and would drink large amounts of water and chew gum to beat the sensation, which left him feeling "joyful for being in control." Other times he would eat vicariously by treating others to gourmet dinners, while not eating any food himself. He would spend hours reading cookbooks and food magazines, all while resisting his severe hunger pangs.

My first action was to acknowledge that Russell would make his own decisions about when to eat, but I also said that going hungry was not a positive achievement. I explained the serious physical ramifications of continuing his behavior. We spent some time eliciting Russell's personal long-term wishes: get married, take over the family business, and several other future-oriented goals. With this leverage and his expressed agreement, we then spent some time discussing the destructive medical consequences that he could expect if he continued his anorectic and bulimic behaviors. This was a revelation as, surprisingly, he had never been informed of such effects as osteoporosis, kidney failure, heart failure, and mental health problems. We then addressed how to stop his laxative abuse. This goal was important because he had tried to stop abusing laxatives on occasion but had experienced serious constipation and other side effects such as stomach cramps and loss of energy. Consequently, he quickly resumed his laxative abuse. We also discussed how to control his exercise regimen.

I also addressed Russell's severe dehydration. I informed him that when he began to hydrate adequately, he might experience sudden fluctuations in body weight that would be due to fluid changes in his body, not a sudden gain in fat. Additionally, he gradually increased his energy intake by approximately 50 kcal per day (209 kJ per day), beginning with high-quality protein sources and eventually a variety of other foods. Russell continued to attend regular sessions with me over the next 6 months, gradually gaining understanding of the importance of proper nutrition and a normal dietary pattern. I continuously provided Russell with more tools on how to facilitate permanent, positive behavior change. Russell has managed to regain 25 lb (11.4 kg) and learned to accept his body weight as healthy. He has since completed his undergraduate education with honors.

May May Leung, MS, RD
Doctoral Student
University of North Carolina at Chapel Hill

Female Runner With Anorexia Nervosa and Bulimia Nervosa

M.V. is a 22-year-old recreational runner who presented with a clinical eating disorder at our sports medicine facility. Her height was 63 in. (160 cm), and she weighed 110 lb (50 kg). M.V. had a history of anorexia nervosa, but the disorder remained undiagnosed and she sought no treatment at the time. Her lowest body weight was 89 lb (40.4 kg), and her highest body weight was 130 lb (59 kg). During the past 12 months, M.V. engaged in pathological weight-control methods that ranged from severe restriction to binge eating and purging, or bulimia nervosa.

Although building trust is important in a first consultation, the focus should be on assessing warning signs and symptoms important for diagnosis and addressing immediate nutritional and health risks. M.V. reported secondary amenorrhea, having no menstrual cycle for over 12 months. She also complained about depressive symptoms, dizziness during exercise and work, and occasional anemia. Most important, M.V. was highly unstable and extremely judgmental about her bulimic behaviors and her body in general. At the time she presented to our clinic, her binge–purge cycles (using vomiting as purging method) occurred at a rate of three to six times per day and had persisted for longer than 6 months. Thus, she had clinical bulimia nervosa.

Her exercise schedule was intense. She ran 7 to 8 mi (11 to 13 km) per day at a pace of 7:30 per mi (5:40 per km). She performed longer, slower runs on the weekends. M.V. used exercise both to improve her conditioning and to control her weight. She was not a competitive runner, but her goal was to become one. Her daily routine consisted of waking up at 4:00 a.m., going for her run, and then doing 45 minutes of Pilates and other types of strengthening exercises. M.V. worked in landscaping and thus was highly active during her 8 to 10 hr workdays. Several methods were used to assess her total daily energy expenditure, which was estimated to be between 2,800 and 3,500 kcal per day (between 11,704 and 14,630 kJ per day).

Her dietary intake at the time of presentation to our clinic was erratic, with little consistency but multiple large binges per day. Binge foods included sweets (frozen yogurt, ice cream, yogurt, candy, cookies, and desserts) and salty snacks (crackers, chips). Foods that triggered binge eating were similar. A general fear of carbohydrate was also noted, especially regarding starchy foods such as rice, pasta, potatoes, cereals, and bread.

Therapeutic Goals

Here are the therapeutic goals that we established and the strategies used to progress toward them:

1. Decrease nutritional risk and purging frequency and then decrease bingeing.
   - M.V. was initially seen every other day.
   - She began therapy with a psychologist who specialized in eating disorders.
   - A physician monitored her regularly.
2. Provide a structured meal plan.
   - M.V. received a structured meal plan that directed her to eat at specific times and in specific amounts, quantified with household measures.
   - The plan included three meals and three snacks (morning, afternoon, and evening).
   - Portion sizes remained small, except for vegetables.
   - The plan included easily consumable foods.
   - Fear of carbohydrate was initially circumvented by including greater servings of vegetables (including starchy vegetables such as corn, peas, carrots, squash, pumpkin, beets).
   - A journal was encouraged but not required. M.V. wrote in a journal to monitor her emotions when triggered to binge.
   - She was asked to monitor her hunger and satiety for meals and snacks.

3. Address exercise routine.

- Initially, the exercise routine was kept constant except that 1 day was set aside for complete rest.
- After 2 weeks of treatment, running mileage was decreased, but intensity remained constant.
- M.V. continued to receive information, started during her initial consultation, about the dangers of eating disorders, the female athlete triad, and the long-lasting effects of such behaviors.
- Each session included reassessment, reestablishing goals, and education (focused on resolving the many myths about exercise and body weight).
- Work on body image was also incorporated.

Progress

M.V. reduced binge–purge cycles to less than two times per week after 4 weeks of treatment. A temporary injury to her shin caused relapsing problems. M.V. recognized through careful illustration of her compulsive exercise patterns by the sports dietitian that she needed to normalize her volume and intensity. She began to acknowledge that her work as a landscaper could be viewed as a workout on certain days, and she incorporated changes that helped reduce the overload on her shin. With each consultation, an attempt was made to integrate new but "safe" foods into her meal plan. Much work was also dedicated to understanding normal portion sizes and the importance of including small portions of desserts and other challenging foods to reduce the risk of bingeing on those foods later. The psychologist worked intensely in conjunction with the treatment team and not only helped reinforce dietary changes but also focused on the origin of her eating disorder and the incorporation of coping and problem-solving skills.

After the 1st month, consultation was reduced to a weekly schedule. Although the physician had prescribed an antidepressant medication much earlier, M.V. finally began taking it. Recurrent issues with body image and "feeling tight in clothing" made achieving progress difficult. As education focused more on mindful eating and using her coping skills to reduce bingeing, positive results began to occur. M.V.'s body weight fluctuated between 110 to 120 lb (50 to 54.5 kg) during treatment, but as she reduced bingeing, M.V. mentioned several times that she felt more comfortable about her body, that she felt more toned, and that her clothing fit better. This change in outlook coincided with her openness to integrating trigger foods (adding rice and desserts in small quantities) and going out to eat. Surprisingly, she resumed a normal menstrual cycle.

M.V. is still in treatment today, being seen once per month. Her eating disorder patterns have not fully resolved, but she has succeeded in reducing her health and nutritional risk, maintaining a normal menstrual cycle, which she monitors regularly, and performing a more balanced exercise routine. The largest improvement for M.V. was that she increased her dietary intake using consistent meals and snacks, learned about the importance of feeling hunger and satiety, realized the value of being present while preparing and eating food, and most of all came to understand that overeating and bingeing would offer only temporary relief for her emotional imbalances.

Nanna L. Meyer, PhD, RD
Sports Dietitian and Physiologist
The Orthopedic Specialty Hospital (TOSH)
Salt Lake City, Utah

Exercise in
Extreme Environments

This chapter focuses on the athlete or exerciser who exercises in extreme environments, either extreme weather or high altitude. Training and nutrition are both crucial to peak performance in these environments.

PHYSIOLOGICAL CHANGES IN EXTREME ENVIRONMENTS

An extreme environment is one in which the temperature is hot (above 80 °F, or 26.7 °C), especially when accompanied by high humidity, the temperature is cold (below 32 °F, or 0 °C), or the altitude is above 5,280 ft (1,609 m) (Gore Trail Condominiums, 2002). This chapter will cover these three environments.

Although the body constantly produces heat, it produces far more heat during physical exertion. The body passes the heat that it produces to the environment, but when exercising in extreme environmental conditions, the body may not be as adept at dissipating heat as it normally is.

Here is how Survival IQ (2003) describes the four ways that the body can gain or lose heat from the environment:

- Conduction—the transfer of heat from a warm object to a cool one that is touching it. (Warming boots by putting them on is an example.)

- Convection—the transfer of heat by circulation or movement of air. (Using a fan on a hot day is an example.)
- Radiation—the transfer of heat by electromagnetic waves. (Sitting under a heat lamp is an example.)
- Evaporation—the transfer of heat by changing a liquid into a gas. (Evaporating sweat cooling the skin is an example.)

Reprinted from www.survivaliq.com/physical_fitness/enviornmental-considerations_12-1.htm and based on US Army Field Manual 21-20.

Heat and Humidity

Heat moves from warm to cool areas, and during exercise the temperature of the body rises. Under normal conditions, to prevent hyperthermia, the body loses heat by one of the mechanisms mentioned. Nonetheless, sweating is the body's best mechanism for dissipating heat.

Because evaporation rate is inversely related to humidity, the ability of the body to dissipate heat through sweat decreases in hot and humid conditions. Overheating can result, which in turn can lead to heat illness such as muscle (heat) cramps, exercise (heat) exhaustion, heat syncope, exertional hyponatremia, or heatstroke. Table 9.1 provides definitions and causes of each of these types of heat illnesses. Heat illnesses are more likely to occur in those who have not acclimatized to the heat or who have not properly hydrated themselves, regardless of their fitness levels. Note that although heat illnesses mostly occur in hot and humid conditions, they can occur under other conditions as well (Binkley, Beckett, Casa, Kleiner, & Plummer, 2002).

Fit people can acclimatize to hot, humid conditions in 1 to 2 weeks. Someone who is not fit will need more time to acclimatize. Some of the physiological changes that occur with acclimatization are that the body begins to sweat sooner and more profusely, plasma volume increases to cool the body more quickly (an adaptation that also occurs when a person becomes more fit), and the heart rate will be lower at any work intensity (Survival IQ, 2003).

Note that the word *acclimatization* refers to the usual situation in which people exercise in a given environment and their bodies adapt physiologically. *Acclimation*, however, is achieved in an artificial environment, such as a thermal chamber that one might use to train artificially in hot and humid conditions (Sutton, 1996). Although the body will adapt to both environments equally well, the terms should not be used interchangeably.

Cold

In general, exercising in the cold poses less danger than exercising in the heat, although without taking proper precautions, hypothermia, frostbite, and dehydration can ensue (Survival IQ, 2003). If the body drops below its normal temperature of 98.6 °F (37 °C), normal metabolism or bodily function do not occur, a condition known as hypothermia. The body is unable to produce heat as quickly as it is dissipating heat, which can eventually be fatal (Casa, 2002). Under cold conditions, body heat is lost by radiation

Table 9.1   Definitions and Causes of Heat-Related Illnesses

Heat illness	Definition	Causes
Muscle (heat) cramp	Acute, painful, involuntary muscle contraction that occurs during or after exercise.	Dehydration, electrolyte imbalances, neuromuscular fatigue (or combination). Some warning signs of dehydration are tiredness or exhaustion, inability to eat, red skin, heat intolerance, lightheadedness, dark urine with a strong odor.
Exercise (heat) exhaustion	Inability to continue exercise, with any combination of heavy sweating, dehydration, sodium loss, or energy depletion.	Hot, humid conditions (most often); need rectal temperature to distinguish from heat stroke; pallor, persistent muscle cramps; weakness, dizziness, headache, need to defecate; core body temperature between 97 °F (36.1 °C) and 104 °F (40 °C).
Heat syncope	Also called orthostatic dizziness; exposure to high environmental temperatures; occurs during first 5 days of acclimatization or in people with heart disease or taking diuretics.	Peripheral vasodilation, postural pooling of blood, dehydration, decreased cardiac output, decreased venous return, cerebral ischemia; usually occurs after standing for long periods, immediately postexercise, or upon standing after sitting for a long period.
Exertional hyponatremia	Relatively rare; occurs when blood sodium levels go below 130 mmol per L. Typically occurs during bouts of exercise that exceed 4 hours.	Drinking too much low-solute beverage beyond sweat losses (water intoxication) or not replacing sweat sodium losses.
Exertional heat stroke	Elevated core temperature >104 °F (40 °C), with signs of organ system failure because of hyperthermia. Result of excessive heat production by the body or lack of heat dissipation in extreme environmental conditions. Can be life threatening or fatal.	Tachycardia, hypotension, sweating, hyperventilation, altered mental state, vomiting, diarrhea, seizures, coma.

Data from H.M. Binkley (2002), Casa (2002), and Hargreaves (1996).

and convection (Burruss, Castellani, Rundell, & Snyder, 1998). The body produces heat by resting metabolism, the thermic effect of food (also called dietary induced thermogenesis), and muscle contraction (Burruss et al.). Heat production during exercise is 10 to 20 times greater than heat production at rest.

Exposure to the cold, especially if a person is not properly dressed and hydrated, can lead to hypothermia, especially in those who are not acclimatized, but it can occur in people who are acclimatized if they are not properly prepared (dressed, hydrated, and so on). Symptoms of hypothermia include muscle weakness, shivering, impaired speech, loss of judgment, and sleepiness (Survival IQ, 2003).

So how does the body respond to the cold to decrease the effects of hypothermia? The first is shivering thermogenesis (Burruss et al., 1998), in which the body produces heat by involuntary muscle contraction. The body also responds to cold by peripheral vasoconstriction, which decreases blood flow to the skin (Burruss et al.). Combined, these two mechanisms help preserve heat within the body by increased heat production (shivering thermogenesis) and decreased heat lost (peripheral vasoconstriction) (Burruss et al.). Ventilation and heart rate usually increase slightly in cold weather. Furthermore, cold air is typically dryer than hot air. Therefore, maintaining hydration is important because respiratory water loss in cold weather increases through greater water vapor loss. When a person can see his or her breath on a cold day, what is visible is the heat and water vapor that are exhaled from the body. The faster and deeper that a person breathes, as will occur with exercise, the more moisture and heat that the person loses (Burruss et al.).

Proper clothing and hydration are essential to preventing hypothermia. A person exercising in the cold should wear clothing that will cover as much as the body as possible, leaving little skin exposed to the cold air. Wearing layers offers the advantage of allowing the person to remove or add clothing as needed. Buying clothing that breathes and wicks away sweat prevents moisture from remaining close to the body. A cotton T-shirt is not a good choice in cold weather because cotton does not wick away sweat. The head and neck should be covered, because about 40% of heat is lost from the head and neck (Survival IQ, 2003). Hydrating before, during, and after exercise is important, as always (see table 9.2 for a hydration schedule).

Frostbite, the freezing of body tissue (Survival IQ, 2003), occurs most commonly in the nose, ears, feet, and hands. The greater the windchill factor, the greater the risk of getting frostbite. Frostbite can be so severe that amputation may be necessary. To prevent frostbite, people must wear proper clothing, cover as many body parts as possible, and hydrate properly.

High Altitude

Exercising at altitudes below 5,000 ft (1,524 m) typically will not adversely affect a healthy person. At altitudes greater than 5,000 feet above sea level, atmospheric pressure is noticeably lower. Therefore, the body will get less oxygen than it does at sea level (Survival IQ, 2003). Because of the lack of oxygen, both exercise and activities of daily living are much more difficult,

Table 9.2 Hydration Guidelines Based on the 2007 American College Sports Medicine Position Stand on Exercise and Fluid Replacement

When to drink fluids?	Timing	Amount of water or sports drink
Before exercise	At least 4 h before	"Slowly" approximately 5 to 7 mL/kg of body weight*
During exercise	*Ad libitum* (or every 15 to 20 min)	0.4 to 0.8 L of fluid per h** (general guidelines)
After exercise	Up until 2 h post-exercise (or longer, if needed)	1.5 L of fluid/kg of body weight lost

*If the athlete is not producing uring or her urine is dark, ACSM recommends that she consume more fluid in the amount of 3 to 5 mL/kg of body weight.

**A more accurate marker is that fluid replacement during exercise should be approximately equal to sweat and urine losses.

From American College of Sports Medicine, 2007, "Exercise and fluid replacement: Position stand," *Med. Sci. Sports Exercise.* 39(2): 377-390.

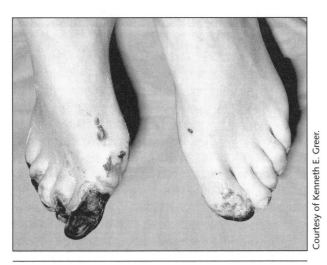

The consequences of failing to dress properly for cold weather exercise, or to take safety precautions such as avoiding wilderness situations for which one is not trained, can be devastating, as this image of frostbite damage illustrates.

especially for those who are unfit, are older, or have chronic illnesses. Nonetheless, the longer a person remains at high altitude, the better his or her exercise performance becomes as acclimatization begins to take effect. Acclimatization can take about 2 weeks, although the time required varies from person to person. Before people become acclimatized, they may suffer from tachycardia, increased heart rate, decreased appetite, nausea, insomnia, and headache (Survival IQ, 2003). A person deacclimatizes in about 2 weeks after returning to sea level (Survival IQ).

Specific physiological changes that occur with high-altitude training include increased ventilation, increased heart rate and cardiac output, and maximum oxygen extraction at the tissue level (Sutton, 1993). When acclimatization begins, the number of red blood cells (and hence the amount of hemoglobin) increases per unit volume of blood, mainly because of a decrease in plasma volume (hemoconcentration) rather than increased production of red blood cells (erythropoiesis) (Sutton, 1993). Other physiological changes induced by acclimatization to high altitude resemble those that occur when a person becomes more fit. For example, major enzymes involved in aerobic metabolism increase, as do the capillary and mitochondrial densities in muscle (Green, Sutton, Young, Cymerman, & Houston, 1989, MacDougall et al., 1991). Unfortunately, the latter changes to capillary and mitochondria densities are due to loss of

muscle mass, not an absolute increase in these parameters (MacDougall et al.).

NUTRITION

This section discusses specific nutritional concerns for those who exercise in extreme environments. In particular, we focus on the effects of heat and humidity, cold, and high altitude on nutritional needs.

Heat and Humidity

Good nutrition should be practiced all the time, of course. Athletes who train and exercise in the heat must pay particular attention to hydration. Exercising in the heat requires the body to adapt to several major physiological changes that occur at one time. These changes affect cardiovascular equilibrium, thermoregulatory maintenance, and muscular power (Murray, 1996). Dehydration added to these circumstances increases a person's chances of contracting a heat illness.

Even a seemingly minor shortfall in hydration can decrease exercise performance; a 2% loss of body weight impairs the cardiovascular system, thermoregulatory response, and exercise endurance. Because dehydration can significantly affect exercise performance, athletes must consume an amount of fluid close to the amount of sweat that they lose (Murray, 1996, 2002). Carbohydrate ingestion along with fluid ingestion can help conserve muscle glycogen and further aid performance. Overhydration is not beneficial and in some cases can result in hyponatremia. A good way for people to discover whether they are consuming the proper amount of fluid is to weigh themselves before and after exercise. Then, by noting the amount of fluid required to return to preexercise weight, they can estimate their fluid requirements during exercise.

Cold

Fluid consumption is a key consideration in exercising in the cold, as it is in heat and humidity. The exerciser should match fluid loss with fluid intake. Another factor to consider is that energy requirements may be greater during exercise in the cold. Thus, a person needs to evaluate overall energy expenditure during workouts to determine whether he or she will require more energy intake.

Courtesy of Kenneth E. Greer.

Sample Meal Plan for People Who Exercise in Extreme Environments

Although it depends on the amount of exercise that a person performs, in most extreme environments additional energy will be required—especially at high altitude and in cold weather. Hydration is also important. Hydration with water or a sports drink that provides from 5% to 7% of energy from carbohydrate is recommended. Increasing salt consumption will help with hydration status.

This sample meal plan provides a guide for those who exercise in extreme environments. Each client must be treated individually, based on the particular extreme environment in which he or she is physically active, as well as the person's gender, training intensity and duration, food likes and dislikes, allergies, and so on.

Breakfast
- 1 1/2 cups of Grape Nuts cereal = 165 g
- 1 cup of skim milk = 240 ml
- 1 cup of strawberries = 230 g
- 1 cup of orange juice = 240 ml
- Water or sports drink, as needed

Snack
- 1 medium orange = 80 g
- 1 medium apple = 80 g
- 1/2 cup of salted mixed nuts = 60 g
- Water or sports drink, as needed

Lunch
- Lean roast beef sandwich (1 1/2 sandwiches)
  - 6 oz of unprocessed sliced roast beef = 180 g
  - 3 slices of whole-wheat bread = 120 g
  - 3 slices of lettuce = 25 g
  - 6 slices of tomato = 120 g
  - 2 tbsp of mayonnaise or mustard = 30 g
- 1 cup of mixed greens salad = 113 g
- 4 tbsp of vinaigrette dressing = 60 g
- 2 cups of skim milk = 480 ml
- Water or sports drink, as needed

Snack
- 8 oz of low-fat strawberry yogurt = 230 g
- 8 double squares of graham crackers = 100 g
- Water or sports drink, as needed

Dinner
- 6 oz of baked salmon = 180 g
- 1 cup of brown rice = 230 g
- 1 cup of steamed kale = 225 g
- 1 cup of steamed sugar snap peas = 230 g
- 2 whole-wheat dinner rolls = 160 g
- 3 tsp of butter or margarine = 15 g
- 2 cups of skim milk = 480 g

Snack
- 1 cup of pretzels = 220 g
- 8 oz of low-fat vanilla yogurt = 230 g
- 1 medium peach = 80 g
- 1 medium banana = 80 g
- Water or sports drink, as needed

Salt intake is encouraged for hydration purposes and to minimize muscle cramping.

This sample meal plan provides at least 100% of the Dietary Reference Intakes (DRIs) for energy, protein, fiber, vitamins A, C, E, B_6, B_{12}, thiamin, riboflavin, niacin, folate, calcium, iron, magnesium, phosphorus, zinc, and approximately

- 3,500 kcal (14,630 kJ),
- 160 g of protein,
- 130 g of fat,
- 38 g of fiber, and
- 5,500 mg of sodium (or more, depending on amount of salt that the person uses at the table).

From S.L. Volpe, S.B. Sabelawski, and C.R. Mohr, 2007, *Fitness nutrition for special dietary needs* (Champaign, IL: Human Kinetics).

High Altitude

Taking in adequate nutrition at high altitudes can be difficult because athletes often do not have the same appetite that they do at sea level. Nonetheless, once acclimatized, the athlete's appetite should return. First, energy intake needs to be increased, and protein intake should be increased slightly because of the loss in muscle mass that usually accompanies high-altitude training. Baseline energy needs may increase by 500 kcal per day (2,090 kJ per day) or more, depending on energy expenditure with training. Resting metabolic rate increases when an athlete first arrives at high altitude (Butterfield et al., 1992).

Hydration is another key factor in nutrition at high altitudes. Athletes need to keep well hydrated and may consider consuming a sports drink with a 5% to 7% carbohydrate concentration to provide some energy. Table 9.2 provides guidelines, although greater fluid intake may be required in some circumstances.

PHYSICAL ACTIVITY

Exercising in extreme environments can be dangerous if acclimatization does not occur. Acclimatization requires training in the relevant conditions and consuming a diet that will maintain energy balance. In addition, proper clothing and equipment are required.

Heat and Humidity

The ability to exercise declines in the heat. Therefore, exercise intensity should be decreased in the heat, at least for the first several days during acclimatization (Maughan & Shirreffs, 1997). Furthermore, training should occur in the cooler parts of the day—early morning is best, but evening can also be a good time to exercise during hot weather. Exercising at those times of day will minimize the possibility of heat illnesses while allowing the athlete to acclimatize. Although the athlete need not exercise every day in the heat (outside rather than working out in a cooler environment indoors), exercising in the heat every 3rd day for 30 days resulted in acclimatization equal to exercising in the heat every day for 10 days (Fein, Haymes, & Buskirk, 1975). Physiological changes occurring in those who have become well acclimatized to hot, humid conditions can

Myths About Using Salt Pills in Hot, Humid Conditions

In the past, when athletes and soldiers engaged in strenuous physical activity in hot, humid conditions, salt pills were provided to help them avoid losing water and salt. This practice is not recommended and can be extremely dangerous! As discussed earlier, acclimatization is essential. Moreover, during and after acclimatization, adequate hydration is required to prevent a heat-related illness from occurring. Salt pills, if they are going to be taken, must be given by a qualified health professional (for example, a physician or registered dietitian) and administered with enough water that the person will not suffer from the consequences of consuming a high dose of salt without fluids in hot, humid conditions. Whatever the conditions, especially in extreme conditions, proper food and fluid intake before, during, and after exercise is essential for good performance and health.

persist for 21 days in a cool environment (Pichan, Sridharan, Swamy, Joseph, & Gautam, 1985).

Although it has been reported that acclimatization occurs best with exercise of 60 to 100 minutes at moderate intensity, exercising 30 minutes per day at about 75% of maximal oxygen consumption ($\dot{V}O_2$max) was as effective for acclimatization as was exercising for 60 minutes per day at 50% of $\dot{V}O_2$max (Houmard et al., 1990). Furthermore, exercising in the heat for longer than 100 minutes offers no clear advantage; that is, greater exposure does not result in more rapid acclimatization (Lind & Bass, 1963).

The intensity of the training should be kept lower for about 3 to 10 days, depending on the athlete. Heat acclimatization takes about 10 to 14 days, although this varies among individuals.

Warming up before exercising in the heat should not unduly increase body temperature (as is the goal for cold-weather warm-ups). The athlete should not wear a lot of clothing during the warm-up or exercise period, should drink plenty of fluids, should take frequent rest breaks, and should warm up and cool down in the shade (Maughan & Shirreffs, 1997).

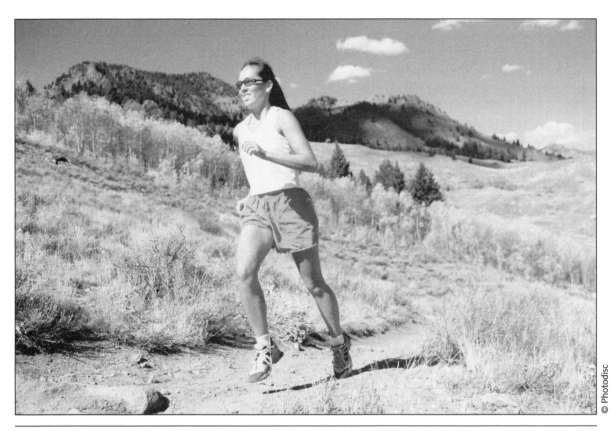

This young woman is putting herself at serious risk for dehydration. She should be carrying water.

Acclimatization does not mean that fluid needs decrease. The opposite happens—with greater acclimatization, the athlete needs more fluids because the sweating response has increased (Maughan & Sherriffs, 1997). Dehydration will lead to impairment in the acclimatization process (Sawka & Pandolf, 1990).

To prevent a person from encountering heat illness, instruct him or her to do the following:

- Have a complete medical examination to evaluate history and risk factors for heat illness.
- Be well trained before exercising in hot and humid conditions.
- Observe healthy nutritional habits, including proper hydration.
- Check environmental conditions (temperature and humidity) and modify the intensity, duration, and frequency of workouts as necessary to reduce risk.
- Take frequent planned water or sports drink breaks during exercise.
- Watch for signs of heat illness.

- Avoid extensive training in hot, humid environments.
- Obtain prompt medical care when unusual responses to exercise in the heat occur.

Adapted from R.B. Kreider, 2003, "The role of Ephedra in the death of a professional baseball player," Center for Exercise, Nutrition & Preventive Health Research, Baylor University.

Cold

Exercise training in the cold also requires adaptation, but typically not to the degree required for exercising in the heat and humidity. That is, the body acclimatizes somewhat to the cold, but not to the extent that it does to hot conditions (Burruss et al., 1998). Nonetheless, exercising in the cold poses some risks, notably frostnip and frostbite. The risk of frostbite is small when the windchill factor is above –20 °F (–28.9 °C). Below that level, the risk increases when skin is exposed (Burruss et al.). As stated earlier, the person exercising in cold conditions should expose as little skin as possible, wear clothes that breathe, and remove wet clothing as soon as possible because wet clothing reduces the insulative properties of

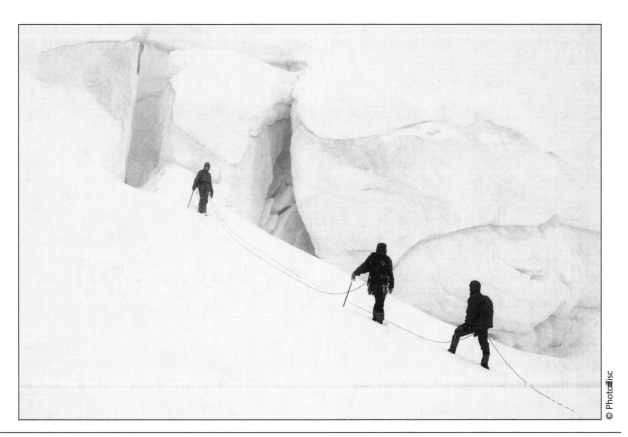

These hikers have dressed wisely for the conditions in which they are exercising. To further ensure their safety, they should all be carrying cell phones close to their bodies to keep the batteries warm and fully functioning.

clothes (Burruss et al.). Interestingly, water is a highly efficient conductor of heat, more than 25 times better than air (Burruss et al.). Wearing gear that protects from wind and rain or snow is important; therefore, waterproof yet breathable clothing is recommended. The athlete may want to exercise with another person, especially if the exercise bout is in a remote place, to permit a quicker response should a problem occur. If possible, the person should take a cellular phone for added precaution.

High Altitude

A person may feel nauseated when beginning to train at high altitudes. Therefore, during the first few days at high altitude, a person may want to do minimal physical activity and allow his or her body to acclimatize a bit. After a few days, the person should start exercising at low intensity and for short bouts several times during the day, if possible. If that schedule is not possible, then exercising for a short bout in the morning and then again in the evening early on will help with acclimatization. Over time, the person can

Prescribing Exercise for Extreme Environments

In this chapter, we discussed how a person should become acclimatized to heat, humidity, cold, and high altitude. Although far less acclimatization occurs to the cold than it does to the heat, some does take place. In general, for all these conditions, a person should start slowly, at an intensity lower than that to which he or she is accustomed. This approach will allow acclimatization to occur, which may take up to 2 weeks in hot, humid conditions and at high altitude. Exercising daily will speed up acclimatization. In extremely hot environments, exercising during the cooler part of the day, at shorter-than-accustomed duration, and lower-than-usual intensity early on is safest. The athlete can then gradually increase duration and intensity while moving to the hotter times of the day. With high-altitude training, the athlete may want to do minimal training at first until he or she overcomes the side effects of the altitude. Then, a gradual increase in exercise duration and intensity can take place over time.

increase duration and then intensity of the exercise bouts.

CASE STUDY

This client came to me through casual conversation when I was discussing sports nutrition with another group. He is an avid cyclist who participates in the Ride the Rockies tour each year, which consists of cycling more than 400 mi (650 km) through the mountains of Colorado. He is paraplegic.

From his dietary recall he demonstrated good intake of protein, carbohydrate, and healthy fat, and his energy intake is adequate. His body weight was estimated at 150 lb (68 kg). He came to me complaining of chronic diarrhea during the tour. In reviewing his intake during the week of the tour, he disclosed that he drank "greens" to maintain his energy throughout the tour. He explained that his energy level was great but that he suffered from diarrhea. This problem resulted from the high fiber content of the greens powder (spirulina powder) that he was taking, which he typically mixed in juice. I explained that the fiber content was probably causing him to have diarrhea.

Because he had a good knowledge base of healthy foods, I did not have to make drastic changes in his day-to-day plan. I discussed the types of sugar that would work best for long endurance events and suggested that he try a few different products until he found one that worked well. In addition, I emphasized the importance of testing beforehand all foods and beverages that he planned to consume during the tour to assess whether they caused gastrointestinal upset. I provided him with information about tapering his fiber intake during the week or so before the tour and provided him with examples of different products that would help him maintain his energy level during the tour. I stressed the importance of recovery nutrition and explained that he would not have adequate energy if his recovery nutrition plan was not in place before the start of the tour.

We worked together to get him through the tour, and I am happy to report that he had no gastrointestinal problems after making the small changes that I suggested. He maintained his energy level throughout the entire tour and is already planning next year's ride.

Mona R. Treadwell, MS, RD

Medical Account Manager for Healthetech

HealtheTech, Inc.

Denver, Colorado

Afterword: Summary and Future Research Recommendations

In this book, we have discussed nutrition that is beneficial for exercisers at different stages of life and in various health conditions. Chapters 1 and 2 dealt with the important role that nutrition and exercise play in the lives of children, adolescents, and older adults. Chapters 3 and 4 covered fitness nutrition for menopause and pregnancy. In chapter 5 we covered vegetarian athletes, and in chapter 6 we discussed active people and athletes who require weight management. In chapter 7 we took a comprehensive look at diabetes mellitus. In chapter 8 we covered eating disorders and disordered eating, and finally, in chapter 9, we wrapped up with fitness nutrition for extreme environments.

We hope that this book helped you with your practice and will continue to do so. The book may have even helped you personally. We believe that nutrition and exercise, combined with proper sleep, a supportive social network, and positive attitudes, can give people healthier and better lives. We also believe in individualizing nutrition and exercise prescriptions for each person. Because people differ significantly from one another, the sample exercise prescriptions and menus are to be used as a guide, not as one-size-fits-all "recipes." It is also important to realize that the more we know about nutrition and exercise, the more questions we have. Thus, we offer our ideas for future research efforts below:

Exercise and nutrition for children and adolescents need to be studied more. Because of the large number of children who are now competing in sports at an early age, more research needs to be conducted on the nutrition needs of children who exercise at high intensity. Furthermore, the rate of type 2 diabetes mellitus is increasing in children because of the increase in overweight. Thus, more research is required about children who have diabetes and who exercise as well as on children's needs as they exercise, lose weight, and experience periods of rapid growth.

Our society is becoming older. According to the United States Census Bureau (www.census.gov/prod/www/abs/popula.html), in the year 2030 approximately 20% of the United States population will be 65 years of age or older. Data are similar for countries around the world. For example, in Italy 28.1% of the population will be 65 years of age or older in 2030. China and Canada will have 16.0% and 22.9% of their populations over the age of 65, respectively, in 2030. Because we are living longer, more research is required about the needs of the older people who exercise. In addition, because some older people who exercise may have some form of chronic disease, the combination of age and disease with exercise and nutrition must be considered.

The menopausal years can be difficult for many women; the degree of menopausal symptoms and duration of this transition in life vary. Most research on menopausal and postmenopausal women has focused on preventing bone loss. Although this research is useful, more research needs to be conducted on menopausal women who exercise at higher intensity. More research is required on the interaction of exercise, diet, and menopausal symptoms and the best combination of the three for women who suffer from moderate to severe menopausal symptoms.

Pregnancy is a unique time in a woman's life, and the body undergoes many physiological changes. Some of the changes that result from pregnancy mirror those that occur with exercise, but for different reasons (for example, an increase in cardiac output). A useful approach would be longitudinal research that follows women through pregnancy to assess the effects of exercise in each trimester and evaluate the results of differing exercise intensity among women. Nutritional requirements need to be better defined for those who are pregnant and exercise.

Although a great deal of research has been conducted on vegetarian diets and health and assessment of athletes' diets, little research has been conducted on athletic performance among vegetarian athletes. Many athletes have been extremely successful while eating a vegetarian diet. An assessment of dietary intake among those athletes would be one step in furthering our knowledge about vegetarian diets and high-intensity exercise.

In chapter 6 we discussed exercise, nutrition, and weight management. Although exercise and diet are clearly important for weight loss and management, research is required to assess the needs of people who have lost weight, maintained their weight loss, and continue to exercise frequently, for long durations, or at high intensity. Their needs will change over time, but they may be different from the needs of people who have exercised for a long time but have not experienced weight loss.

The interaction among nutrition, exercise, and diabetes mellitus is an expanding field. New medications for both type 1 and type 2 diabetes mellitus will appear, and they may prove to be more effective and efficient in controlling blood glucose levels and glycosylated hemoglobin. Research is needed on the effects of exercise by those with diabetes, focusing on the number of years of exercise and the type of exercise in preventing long-term complications. This kind of research will help quantify the benefits of exercise and may promote more rapid adjustment of exercise and intake of insulin or medications, as well as nutrition.

In chapter 8 we discussed eating disorders and disordered eating—a topic that can be difficult to discuss with the person who is suffering from one of these disorders. Nonetheless, individuals with eating disorders and disordered eating must be treated promptly. Because overexercise and dysfunctional eating patterns have been the crux of most eating disorders, a person with this kind of disorder needs to learn to exercise and eat in a healthy manner. Research in this area is required to determine the prevalence of disordered eating among males, to discover ways to identify disordered eating in people more quickly, and to educate all athletes, especially female athletes, of the dangers of eating disorders and disordered eating to their performance and overall health.

Finally, the chapter on exercising under extreme conditions—at high altitude, in the cold, or in hot and humid weather—is valuable because all athletes have or will exercise under at least one of these conditions. More research is required to assess the long-term effects of performing physical work, not necessarily physical exercise, in these conditions. For example, what are the effects on people who work in construction or serve in the military? These people work long hours under extreme conditions and thus may have greater vitamin and mineral requirements than those who exercise in extreme conditions for, say, 45 minutes per day.

We have provided you with some ideas for future research, although we could list many more. Please feel free to contact any of us should you have suggestions for future research or revisions (Dr. Stella Lucia Volpe at svolpe@nursing.upenn.edu). We look forward to hearing from you!

Appendix

Table A.1 Carbohydrate Sources

Select most often	Select moderately	Select least often
Amaranth	Cornbread	Brown sugar
Barley	Corn tortillas	Brown rice syrup
Beans	Couscous	Chicory syrup
Brown rice	Grits	Confectioner's sugar
Buckwheat	Noodles	Corn syrup
Bulgur (cracked wheat)	Spaghetti	Dextrose
Millet	Macaroni	Evaporated cane juice
Oatmeal	Most ready-to-eat breakfast cereals	Glucose
Quinoa	Pitas	High-fructose corn syrup
Sorghum	Pretzels	Honey
Triticale	White bread	Malt syrup
Wheat berries	White crackers	Maltodextrin
Whole-grain barley	White flour tortillas	Molasses
Whole-grain cornmeal	White sandwich buns and rolls	Raw sugar
Whole rye	White rice	
Whole-grain bread		
Whole-wheat crackers		
Whole-wheat pasta		
Whole-wheat tortillas		
Wild rice		

Note: This list does not include all suitable food choices.

Table A.2 Protein Sources

Select most often	Select moderately	Select least often
Beans	Canadian bacon	Bacon
Chicken breast (without skin)	Lean cuts of beef or pork	Chicken (with skin)
Crab	Low-fat luncheon meats (e.g., turkey)	Chicken wings
Egg whites	Mixed nuts	Fatty beef, lamb, pork
Flounder	Peanut butter	Fatty luncheon meats (e.g.,
Halibut	Reduced-fat and part-skim cheese	bologna, pastrami, corned beef)
Low-fat or nonfat cottage cheese	Shrimp	Fried chicken and fish
Low-fat or nonfat milk (cow's milk, soy milk, rice milk)	Texturized vegetable protein	Liver
	Turkey bacon	Ribs
Low-fat or nonfat yogurt	Whole eggs	Sausage
Salmon		Turkey (with skin)
Snapper (red or blue)		Untrimmed beef and pork
Soy milk		Whole milk
Tilapia		Whole milk cheese
Tofu		
Tuna (steaks or canned, in water)		
Turkey breast (without skin)		

Note: This list does not include all suitable food choices.

Table A.3 Fat Sources

Select most often	Select moderately	Select least often
Avocado Fish oil Flax oil Mixed nuts Olives Olive oil Soybean oil Sunflower oil Walnut oil	Egg yolks Margarine (without trans fat) Vegetable oil	Animal fat Butter Coconut oil Cream Fried foods Ice cream Lard and shortening Shortening Sour cream Whole-fat dairy products

Note: This list does not include all suitable food choices.

Table A.4 Fruits and Vegetables

Green	Yellow or orange	Blue or purple	White	Red
Artichoke Arugula Asparagus Bok choy Broccoli Brussels sprouts Cabbage Celery Collard greens Cucumber Green beans Green grapes Green peas Green pepper Kale Kiwi Lima beans Mesclun greens Mustard greens Okra Peas Romaine lettuce Spinach Turnip greens Watercress Zucchini	Acorn squash Apricots Butternut squash Cantaloupe (rockmelon) Carrots Corn Grapefruit Lemon Mango Nectarine Orange Papaya Peach Pineapple Pumpkin Sweet potato Yellow squash	Beets Blackberries Black grapes Blueberries Eggplant Elderberries Figs Plums Purple cabbage	Banana Bean sprouts Cauliflower Garlic Kohlrabi Mushroom Onion Parsnip Rutabaga Shallots Turnips Wax beans White potato	Apple Pomegranate Red potato Radish Raspberry Red onion Red pepper Strawberry Tomatoes Tomato juice Watermelon

Eating a variety of fruits and vegetables, including at least one selection from each column (and more than that from at least two more), will ensure consumption of a healthy amount of vitamins and micronutrients.

Note: This list does not include all suitable food choices.

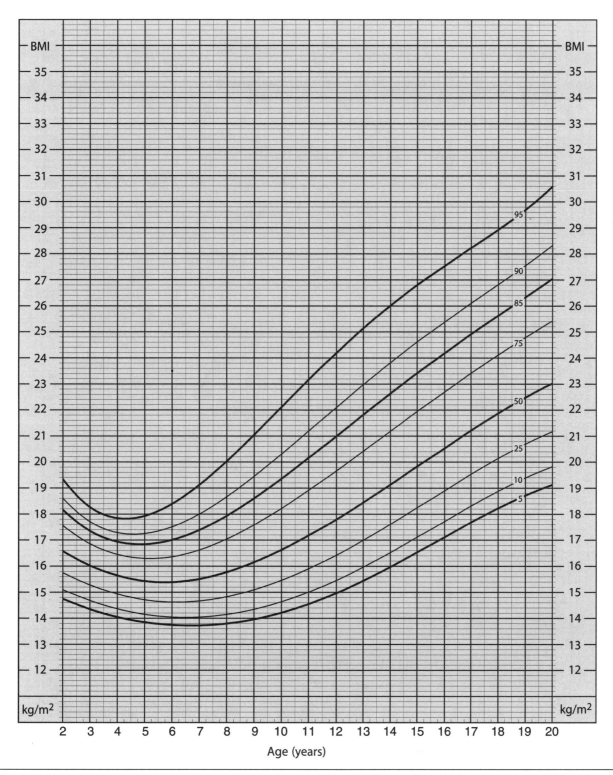

Figure A.1 BMI line graph for boys.

Centers for Disease Control and Prevention, National Center for Health Statistics. CDC growth charts: United States.

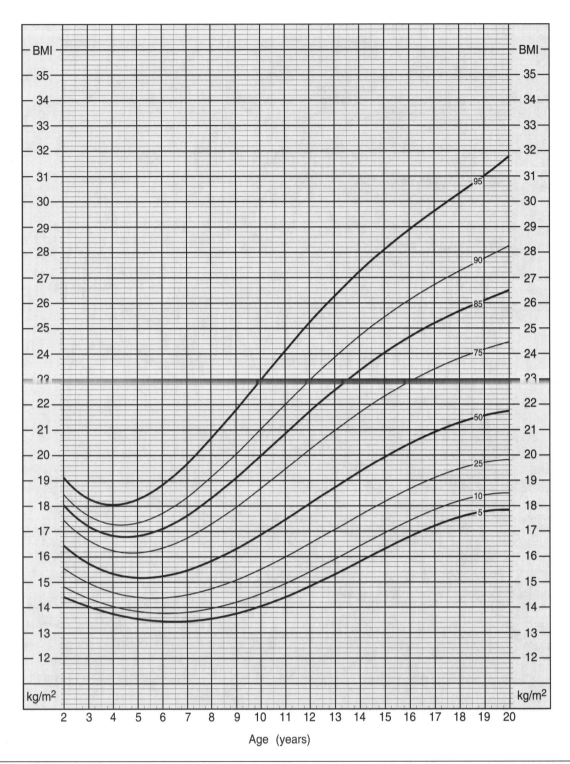

Figure A.2 BMI line graph for girls.

Centers for Disease Control and Prevention, National Center for Health Statistics. CDC growth charts: United States.

Glossary

amenorrhea—Abnormal absence of menses; typically zero to three menstrual cycles per year.

anabolic—A metabolic reaction in which smaller molecules come together to build larger ones, that is, "to build up."

anemia—Deficiency disease in red blood cells, hemoglobin, or total blood volume, typically resulting from iron deficiency. Deficiencies in other nutrients can also cause anemias. For example, a deficiency in folate or vitamin B_{12} can result in megaloblastic anemia.

anorexia nervosa—Eating disorder marked by distorted perception of body weight and refusal to maintain a normal body weight. Anorexia nervosa is a psychological disorder that results in serious adverse physiological changes.

antioxidants—Compounds in some foods, like fruits or vegetables, that guard against oxidation by being oxidized themselves. Oxidation is thought to be one cause of cancer, heart disease, and even aging.

bioavailability—Extent to which a nutrient is absorbed; the greater the bioavailability of a nutrient, the greater the amount of the nutrient that is absorbed.

blood lipid level or profile—List of the blood tests that can predict cardiovascular disease risk factors, which typically include serum total cholesterol, serum low-density lipoprotein cholesterol (LDL-C), serum high-density lipoprotein cholesterol (HDL-C), the ratio of serum total cholesterol to serum HDL-C, the ratio of serum LDL-C to serum HDL-C, and serum triglyceride concentration.

body composition—Amount of muscle tissue, fat tissue, bone mineral density, and other tissues that make up a person's total body weight. Body composition can be measured in various ways, including hydrostatic (or underwater) weighing, dual-energy X-ray absorptiometry (DEXA), or more simply, but less accurately, by skinfold measurements.

body mass index (BMI)—Equation that takes into account a person's body weight (in kg) and height (in cm). BMI = weight (kg)/height (m^2). Higher BMIs (>25) are related to greater risk of chronic diseases, whereas lower BMIs (<18) are related to greater risk of respiratory infections and depressed immune function.

bone mineral density—Assessment of bone mass that makes up the mineral content of the bone, typically expressed as grams of mineral per centimeter of bone.

bulimia nervosa—Eating disorder characterized by repeated bouts of one or more of the following: binge eating followed by self-induced vomiting, laxative abuse, diuretics abuse, fasting, or excessive exercise. The person with bulimia nervosa is typically of normal body weight, so the presence of this eating disorder is difficult to detect.

cachexia—Severe muscle wasting.

cardiovascular disease (CVD)—Nonspecific term for all diseases of the heart and blood vessels. Atherosclerosis and arteriosclerosis are two common causes of CVD.

catabolic—A metabolic reaction in which larger molecules are broken down into smaller ones; that is, "to break down."

comorbidities—Occurrence of one or more diseases or disorders besides the primary disease or disorder.

C-reactive protein (CRP)—Plasma protein indicator that determines the level of internal inflammation. CRP is a strong predictor of coronary heart disease.

diabetes mellitus (DM)—Metabolic disorder of carbohydrate metabolism. Typical symptoms include increased blood glucose levels, usually as a result of insufficient insulin production (type 1 diabetes mellitus) or insufficient ability to utilize insulin (type 2 diabetes mellitus).

diverticular disease—Can be thought of in two phases. When a person is diagnosed with diverticular disease but does not presently have symptoms, the condition is called diverticulosis or condition of diverticula. When a person does have symptoms, such as strong pain in the abdominal region, the condition is called diverticulitis or inflammation of the divericula. Divericula are small pouches that form within the large intestine (colon) as a result of feces accumulating because of lack of fiber intake. The feces can make these pouches, and foodstuffs and feces can become stuck in them, causing inflammation and pain.

dyslipidemia—Abnormal lipid levels, typically indicative of increased cardiovascular disease risk (if the lipid levels are elevated).

essential amino acids—Amino acids that the body is not able to synthesize in adequate amounts to meet the body's needs; these amino acids need to be obtained through dietary sources.

estrogen—Hormones responsible for the menstrual cycle and female characteristics.

ferritin—Storage form of iron in the liver and spleen. Low levels of ferritin indicate low iron storage and often precede iron deficiency anemia.

fiber—Substance found in plant foods that is not recognized by, and therefore not digested by, human digestive enzymes.

follicle stimulating hormone (FSH)—Hormone that promotes maturation of the ovarian follicles in women and sperm production in men.

gallstones—Hardened, stonelike substances that can be formed within the gallbladder or in the bile ducts. Surgical removal of the gallbladder is the usual course of action.

gout—Metabolic disease characterized by inflammation of the joints and typically the presence of an excessive amount of uric acid in the blood.

glycosylated hemoglobin—Percentage of glucose bound to hemoglobin. This measure is a long-term (3-month) indicator of how well a person has controlled his or her blood glucose levels. Normal levels are less than 6%.

hematocrit—Measure of the proportion of blood volume occupied by red blood cells. A person who has a hematocrit of 47% has 47% of his or her blood volume composed of red blood cells.

heme—represents the part of hemoglobin and myoglobin that contains iron. About 40% of iron in animal proteins (e.g., meat, poultry, fish) is related to heme, while the remaining 60% is nonheme iron (Taber, 1989).

hemoglobin—Protein that carries oxygen in the blood, gives blood its red color, and is the primary compound in red blood cells. Low hemoglobin levels are a sign of iron deficiency anemia and can affect exercise performance and activities of daily living.

high-density lipoprotein cholesterol (HDL-C)—Plasma lipoprotein containing a large portion of protein and less cholesterol and triglyceride. High levels of HDL-C are associated with decreased risk of cardiovascular disease. Exercise, weight loss, maintenance of a healthy body weight, and stopping smoking are a few ways to increase HDL-C concentrations.

homocysteine—Amino acid indicative of a risk factor for cardiovascular disease; high homocysteine levels are predictive of cardiovascular disease.

hyperlipidemia—Elevated blood lipid levels.

hypertension—Elevated blood pressure, above 120/80 mmHg. New "prehypertension" blood pressure levels have become a bit stricter because hypertension is known as a silent killer.

hypoalbunemia—Reduction in blood albumin levels (normal levels range from 3.5 to 5.0 g per dl).

hypovolemia—Low blood volume.

indirect calorimetry—Indirect method of assessing metabolic rate, either at rest (basal or resting energy expenditure must be assessed in a fasted state for accurate results), during exercise, or after meal consumption (must be assessed for 4 hours after meal consumption for accurate results of dietary-induced thermogenesis). Thus, indirect calorimetry can provide an estimate of total energy expenditure by assessing basal (or resting) metabolic rate, thermic effect of exercise, and dietary induced thermogenesis, respectively. Indirect calorimetry uses an instrument called a metabolic cart. This cart is able to assess oxygen consumption and carbon dioxide expiration, and from these measures it can calculate energy expenditure.

insulin—Hormone secreted by the pancreas in response to elevated blood glucose concentrations.

intrinsic factor—Substance in the stomach that facilitates vitamin B_{12} absorption.

isoflavones—Class of phytochemicals with estrogen-like activity.

ketoacidosis—Acidosis resulting from elevated ketone bodies in the bloodstream; often seen in uncontrolled diabetes mellitus.

ketone bodies—substances made from the partial metabolism of fat. These are synthesized when too little glucose is available for energy. Often seen in uncontrolled diabetes or in high-protein diets.

ketosis—Elevated ketone bodies in the blood and urine; typically observed in uncontrolled diabetes mellitus.

lean body mass—Total body weight minus the fat content of the body. This term is often used interchangeably with fat-free mass, but true fat-free mass cannot be evaluated unless analyzing a cadaver.

lipolysis—Breakdown of fat.

low-density lipoprotein cholesterol (LDL-C)—Lipoproteins that contain high levels of cholesterol; high levels are linked to increased risk of cardiovascular disease.

macrobiotic diet—Highly restrictive diets limited to only a few foods (for example, grains and vegetables).

macronutrient—Term used to describe the energy-yielding, larger nutrients (carbohydrate, protein, and fat).

megaloblastic anemia—Anemia characterized by large cells. Megaloblastic anemia is a result of folate or vitamin B_{12} deficiency.

menopause—Absence of menses for at least 12 months, usually occurring in women between the ages of 45 and 50 but can begin earlier or later in life.

metabolic syndrome—Combination of risk factors associated with insulin resistance including hypertension, hypercholesterolemia, and obesity.

metabolism—All of the reactions that occur in living beings.

micronutrient—Term used to describe the non-energy-yielding, smaller nutrients (vitamins and minerals).

monounsaturated fat—Made of triglycerides where the fatty acids are primarily monounsaturated; that is, most have only one double bond. Monounsaturated fats have been shown to decrease LDL-C and possibly increase HDL-C.

morbidity—Having a disease.

mortality—State of being dead.

nutrient—Substances obtained from foods and used for energy or various metabolic processes in the body. Two major types of nutrients are macronutrients (i.e., carbohydrates, fats, proteins) and micronutrients (i.e., vitamins and minerals).

nutrient density—Measure of the nutrients that a food provides with respect to the energy it provides. The greater the amount of nutrients and the lower the energy content of a food, the higher its nutrient density.

omega-3 fatty acids—Polyunsaturated fatty acid, designated as such because the first double bond is three carbons away from the methyl end of the carbon.

osteoarthritis—*Osteo* refers to "bone" and *arthritis* refers to "inflammation of the joint"; thus *osteoarthritis* is defined as "inflammation of the bone joint." This painful disease is caused by breakdown of the necessary joint fluids and cartilage.

osteoporosis—Condition in which bones become weak and porous, which typically occurs postmenopausally or in older ages. Osteoporosis can also occur early in life because of amenorrhea or other causes.

oxalates—Found in many vegetables, especially dark leafy green vegetables, and refers to the salt of oxalic acid. High levels of oxalates may form into calcium oxalate stones, or kidney stones.

phytates—Phytic acid is within plant foods, usually the husks of grains, legumes, and seeds, and can chelate with some minerals, decreasing their bioavailability.

phytochemicals—Nonnutrient compounds in plants that have been found to protect against some diseases.

phytoestrogens—Estrogen-like compounds naturally found in plant foods (for example, vegetables and fruits).

polycystic ovary syndrome (PCOS)—Endocrine disturbance associated with primary anovulation and polycystic ovaries.

polyunsaturated fat—Fat that consists of triglycerides in which most of the fatty acids are polyunsaturated; a fat containing at least two double bonds.

prediabetes—Characterized by glucose levels that are higher than normal, yet not high enough to be diagnosed as diabetes mellitus.

preeclampsia—Characterized by hypertension, fluid retention, and protein in the urine; formerly known as pregnancy-induced hypertension.

progesterone—Hormone that is elevated during pregnancy.

saturated fat—Consists mostly of triglycerides that are saturated, having no double bonds.

thermogenesis—Generation of heat; used in physiology and nutrition studies as an index of how much energy the body is using.

References

Chapter 1

Bar-Or, O., IOC Medical Commission, & International Federation of Sports Medicine. (1996). *The child and adolescent athlete*. Oxford: Cambridge, MA.

Beals, K.A. (2004). *Disordered eating among athletes: A comprehensive guide for health professionals*. Champaign, IL: Human Kinetics.

Bellisle, F. (2004). Effects of diet on behaviour and cognition in children. *British Journal of Nutrition, 92*(Suppl. 2), S227–232.

Bolster, D.R., Pikosky, M.A., McCarthy, L.M., & Rodriguez, N.R. (2001). Exercise affects protein utilization in healthy children. *Journal of Nutrition, 131*(10), 2659–2663.

Convertino, V.A., Armstrong, L.E., Coyle, E.F., Mack, G.W., Sawka, M.N., Senay, L.C., Jr., et al. (1996). American College of Sports Medicine position stand. Exercise and fluid replacement. *Medicine and Science in Sports and Exercise, 28*(1), i–vii.

Deurenberg, P., van der Kooy, K., Paling, A., & Withagen, P. (1989). Assessment of body composition in 8-11 year old children by bioelectrical impedance. *European Journal of Clinical Nutrition, 43*(9), 623–629.

Eriksson, B.O. (1972). *Physical training, oxygen supply and muscle metabolism in 11-13-year old boys*. Acta Physiol Scand Suppl. 384, 1–48.

Fagot-Campagna, A. (2000). Emergence of type 2 diabetes mellitus in children: Epidemiological evidence. *Journal of Pediatric Endocrinology and Metabolism, 13*(Suppl. 6), 1395–1402.

Food and Nutrition Board of the Institute of Medicine. (2005). *Dietary Reference Intakes for energy, carbohydrate, fiber, fat, fatty acids, cholesterol, protein, and amino acids (macronutrients)*. Washington, DC: National Academy of Sciences.

Forshee, R.A., & Storey, M.L. (2003). Total beverage consumption and beverage choices among children and adolescents. *International Journal of Food Sciences and Nutrition, 54*(4), 297–307.

Fox, M.K., Devaney, B., Reidy, K., Razafindrakoto, C., & Ziegler, P. (2006). Relationship between portion size and energy intake among infants and toddlers: Evidence of self-regulation. *Journal of the American Dietetic Association, 106*(1 Suppl. 1), S77–S83.

Grantham-McGregor, S., & Ani, C. (2001). A review of studies on the effect of iron deficiency on cognitive development in children. *Journal of Nutrition, 131*(2S-2), 649S–666S; discussion 666S–668S.

Hallberg, L. (1981). Bioavailability of dietary iron in man. *Annual Review of Nutrition, 1*, 123–147.

Haymes, E.M. (1991). Vitamin and mineral supplementation to athletes. *International Journal of Sport Nutrition, 1*(2), 146–169.

Hedley, A.A., Ogden, C.L., Johnson, C.L., Carroll, M.D., Curtin, L.R., & Flegal, K.M. (2004). Prevalence of overweight and obesity among U.S. children, adolescents, and adults, 1999–2002. *Journal of the American Medical Association, 291*(23), 2847–2850.

Ho, C.S., Gould, R.A., Jensen, L.N., Kiser, S.J., Mozar, A., Jensen, J.B. (1991). Evaluation of nutrient content on school, sack and vending lunch of junior high students. *School Food Service Research Review, 15*(2):85–90.

Houtkooper, L.B., Lohman, T.G., Going, S.B., & Hall, M.C. (1989). Validity of bioelectric impedance for body composition assessment in children. *Journal of Applied Physiology, 66*(2), 814–821.

Kennedy, E., & Goldberg, J. (1995). What are American children eating? Implications for public policy. *Nutrition Reviews, 53*(5), 111–126.

Klesges, R.C., Shelton, M.L., & Klesges, L.M. (1993). Effects of television on metabolic rate: Potential implications for childhood obesity. *Pediatrics, 91*(2), 281–286.

Koplan, J.P., Liverman, C.T., & Kraak, V.A. (2005). *Preventing childhood obesity: Health in the balance.* Retrieved December 14, 2005 from www.nap.edu/catalog/11015.html

Littleton, H.L., & Ollendick, T. (2003). Negative body image and disordered eating behavior in children and adolescents: What places youth at risk and how can these problems be prevented? *Clinical Child and Family Psychology Review, 6*(1), 51–66.

Ludwig, D.S., & Ebbeling, C.B. (2001). Type 2 diabetes mellitus in children: Primary care and public health considerations. *Journal of the American Medical Association, 286*(12), 1427–1430.

Lytle, L.A. (2002). Nutritional issues for adolescents. *Journal of the American Dietetic Association, 102*(3 Suppl), S8–12.

Moore, D.C. (1993). Body image and eating behavior in adolescents. *Journal of the American College of Nutrition, 12*(5), 505–510.

Nicklas, T.A. (1995). Dietary studies of children and young adults (1973–1988): The Bogalusa Heart Study. *American Journal of the Medical Sciences, 310 Suppl 1*, S101–108.

Nicklas, T. A., Bao, W., Webber, L.S., & Berenson, G.S. (1993). Breakfast consumption affects adequacy of total daily intake in children. *Journal of the American Dietetic Association, 93*(8), 886–891.

Olshansky, S.J., Passaro, D.J., Hershow, R.C., Layden, J., Carnes, B.A., Brody, J., et al. (2005). A potential decline in life expectancy in the United States in the 21st century. *New England Journal of Medicine, 352*(11), 1138–1145.

Oppliger, R.A., Case, H.S., Horswill, C.A., Landry, G.L., & Shelter, A.C. (1996). American College of Sports Medicine position stand. Weight loss in wrestlers. *Medicine and Science in Sports and Exercise, 28*(6), ix–xii.

Petrie, H.J., Stover, E.A., & Horswill, C.A. (2004). Nutritional concerns for the child and adolescent competitor. *Nutrition, 20*(7–8), 620–631.

Pikosky, M., Faigenbaum, A., Westcott, W., & Rodriguez, N. (2002). Effects of resistance training on protein utilization in healthy children. *Medicine and Science in Sports and Exercise, 34*(5), 820–827.

Pollitt, E., & Mathews, R. (1998). Breakfast and cognition: An integrative summary. *American Journal of Clinical Nutrition, 67*(4), 804S–813S.

Rankinen, T., Fogelholm, M., Kujala, U., Rauramaa, R., & Uusitupa, M. (1995). Dietary intake and nutritional status of athletic and nonathletic children in early puberty. *International Journal of Sport Nutrition, 5*(2), 136–150.

Rivera-Brown, A.M., Gutierrez, R., Gutierrez, J.C., Frontera, W.R., & Bar-Or, O. (1999). Drink composition, voluntary drinking, and fluid balance in exercising, trained, heat-acclimatized boys. *Journal of Applied Physiology, 86*(1), 78–84.

Rodriguez, N.R. (2005). Optimal quantity and composition of protein for growing children. *Journal of the American College of Nutrition, 24*(2), 150S–154S.

Sampson, A.E., Dixit, S., Meyers, A.F., & Houser, R., Jr. (1995). The nutritional impact of breakfast consumption on the diets of inner-city African-American elementary school children. *Journal of the National Medical Association, 87*(3), 195–202.

Shils, M.E. (1999). *Modern nutrition in health and disease* (9th ed.). Baltimore: Williams & Wilkins.

Steen, S.N. (1996a). Timely statement of the American Dietetic Association: Nutrition guidance for adolescent athletes in organized sports. *Journal of the American Dietetic Association, 96*(6), 611–612.

Steen, S.N. (1996b). Timely statement of the American Dietetic Association: Nutrition guidance for child athletes in organized sports. *Journal of the American Dietetic Association, 96*(6), 610–611.

Wardlaw, G.M., Hampl, J.S., & DiSilvestro, R.A. (2004). *Perspectives in nutrition* (6th ed.). Boston: McGraw-Hill Higher Education.

Wilk, B., Yuxiu, H., Bar-Or, O., Wouters, L.J., & Saris, W.H.M. (2002). Effect of hypohydration on aerobic performance of boys who exercise in the heat. *Medicine and Science in Sports and Exercise, 34*, S48.

Chapter 2

Bilderbeck, N., Holdsworth, M.D., Purves, R., & Davies, L. (1981). Changing food habits among 100 elderly men and women in the United Kingdom. *Journal of Human Nutrition and Dietetics, 35*(6), 448–455.

Blumberg, J. (1997). Nutritional needs of seniors. *Journal of the American College of Nutrition, 16*(6), 517–523.

Bonaiuti, D., Shea, B., Iovine, R., Negrini, S., Robinson, V., Kemper, H.C., et al. (2002). Exercise for preventing and treating osteoporosis in postmenopausal women. *Cochrane Database of Systematic Reviews* (3), CD000333.

Campbell, W.W., Crim, M.C., Dallal, G.E., Young, V.R., & Evans, W.J. (1994). Increased protein requirements in elderly people: New data and retrospective reassessments. *American Journal of Clinical Nutrition, 60*(4), 501–509.

Dawson-Hughes, B., Harris, S.S., Rasmussen, H., Song, L., & Dallal, G.E. (2004). Effect of dietary protein supplements on calcium excretion in healthy older men and women. *Journal of Clinical Endocrinology and Metabolism, 89*(3), 1169–1173.

Evans, W.J. (1999). Exercise training guidelines for the elderly. *Medicine and Science in Sports and Exercise, 31*(1), 12–17.

Fiatarone, M.A., O'Neill, E.F., Ryan, N.D., Clements, K.M., Solares, G.R., Nelson, M.E., et al. (1994). Exercise training and nutritional supplementation for physical frailty in very elderly people. *New England Journal of Medicine, 330*(25), 1769–1775.

Fleg, J.L., O'Connor, F., Gerstenblith, G., Becker, L.C., Clulow, J., Schulman, S.P., et al. (1995). Impact of age on the cardiovascular response to dynamic upright exercise in healthy men and women. *Journal of Applied Physiology, 78*(3), 890–900.

Fletcher, R.H., & Fairfield, K.M. (2002). Vitamins for chronic disease prevention in adults: Clinical applications. *Journal of the American Medical Association, 287*(23), 3127–3129.

Food and Nutrition Board of the Institute of Medicine. Panel on Dietary Reference Intakes for Electrolytes and Water. (2004). *Dietary Reference Intakes for water, potassium, sodium, chloride, and sulfate.* Washington, DC: National Academy Press.

Food and Nutrition Board of the Institute of Medicine. Panel on Micronutrients. (2002). *Dietary Reference Intakes for vitamin A, vitamin K, arsenic, boron, chromium, copper, iodine, iron, manganese, molybdenum, nickel, silicon, vanadium, and zinc.* Washington, DC: National Academy Press.

Food and Nutrition Board of the Institute of Medicine. Standing Committee on the Scientific Evaluation of Dietary Reference Intakes. (1997). *Dietary Reference Intakes for calcium, phosphorus, magnesium, vitamin D, and fluoride.* Washington, DC: National Academy Press.

Food and Nutrition Board of the Institute of Medicine. Standing Committee on the Scientific Evaluation of Dietary Reference Intakes; Panel on Folate, Other B Vitamins, and Choline, Subcommittee on Upper Reference Levels of Nutrients. (1998). *Dietary Reference Intakes for thiamin, riboflavin, niacin, vitamin B_6, folate, vitamin B_{12}, pantothenic acid, biotin, and choline.* Washington, DC: National Academy Press.

Heath, G.W., Hagberg, J.M., Ehsani, A.A., & Holloszy, J.O. (1981). A physiological comparison of young and older endurance athletes. *Journal of Applied Physiology, 51*(3), 634–640.

Hughes, V.A., Fiatarone, M.A., Fielding, R.A., Ferrara, C.M., Elahi, D., & Evans, W.J. (1995). Long-term effects of a high-carbohydrate diet and exercise on insulin action in older subjects with impaired glucose tolerance. *American Journal of Clinical Nutrition, 62*(2), 426–433.

Johnson, M.A., Brown, M.A., Poon, L.W., Martin, P., & Clayton, G.M. (1992). Nutritional patterns of centenarians. *International Journal of Aging & Human Development, 34*(1), 57–76.

Joosten, E., van den Berg, A., Riezler, R., Naurath, H.J., Lindenbaum, J., Stabler, S.P., et al. (1993). Metabolic evidence that deficiencies of vitamin B_{12} (cobalamin), folate, and vitamin B_6 occur commonly in elderly people. *American Journal of Clinical Nutrition, 58*(4), 468–476.

Meredith, C.N., Zackin, M.J., Frontera, W.R., & Evans, W.J. (1987). Body composition and aerobic capacity in young and middle-aged endurance-trained men. *Medicine and Science in Sports and Exercise, 19*(6), 557–563.

Pronsky, Z.M. (2004). *Food medication interactions* (13th ed.). Birchrunville, PA: Food-Medication Interactions.

Ryan, A.S. (2000). Insulin resistance with aging: Effects of diet and exercise. *Sports Medicine, 30*(5), 327–346.

Sansevero, A.C. (1997). Dehydration in the elderly: Strategies for prevention and management. *Nurse Practitioner, 22*(4), 41–42, 51–47, 63–66 passim.

Schiffman, S.S. (1997). Taste and smell losses in normal aging and disease. *Journal of the

American Medical Association, 278(16), 1357–1362.

Chapter 3

Altekin, E., Coker, C., Sisman, A.R., Onvural, B., Kuralay, F., & Kirimli, O. (2005). The relationship between trace elements and cardiac markers in acute coronary syndromes. *Journal of Trace Elements in Medicine and Biology, 18*(3), 235–242.

Arjmandi, B.H., Lucas, E.A., Khalil, D.A., Devareddy, L., Smith, B.J., McDonald, J., et al. (2005). One year soy protein supplementation has positive effects on bone formation markers but not bone density in postmenopausal women. *Nutrition Journal, 4*(1), 8.

Bass, J. (2001). Eat to beat menopause: The right nutrients can help you navigate this passage in time. *Natural Health*, October–November [Online journal].

Castro, I.A., Barroso, L.P., & Sinnecker, P. (2005). Functional foods for coronary heart disease risk reduction: A meta-analysis using a multivariate approach. *American Journal of Clinical Nutrition, 82*(1), 32–40.

Food and Nutrition Board. (1997). *Dietary Reference Intakes for calcium, phosphorus, magnesium, vitamin D, and fluoride*. Washington, DC: National Academy Press.

Guyton, A.C., & Hall, J.E. (1996). *Textbook of medical physiology*. Philadelphia: Saunders.

Jakicic, J.M., Winters, C., Lang, W., & Wing, R. (1999). Effects of intermittent exercise and use of home-exercise equipment on adherence, weight loss, and fitness in overweight women. A randomized trial. *Journal of the American Medical Association, 282*, 1554–1560.

Lange-Collett, J. (2002). Promoting health among perimenopausal women through diet and exercise. *Journal of the American Academy of Nurse Practitioners, 14*(4), 172–177.

Melton, L.J. III, Therneau, T.M., Larson, D.R. (1998). Long-term trends in hip fracture prevalence: The influence of hip fracture incidence and survival. *Osteroporosis International, 8*(1): 68–74.

Nakai, M., Black, M., Jeffery, E.H., & Bahr, J.M. (2005). Dietary soy protein and isoflavones: No effect on the reproductive tract and minimal positive effect on bone resorption in the intact female Fischer 344 rat. *Food and Chemical Toxicology, 43*(6), 945–949.

North American Menopause Society. (2002). Management of postmenopausal osteoporosis: Position statement of the North American Menopause Society. *Menopause: The Journal of the North American Menopause Society, 9*(2), 84–101.

Putadechakum, S., Tanphaichitr, V., Leelahagul, P., Pakpeankitvatana, V., Surapisitchart, T., & Komindr, S. (2005). Long-term treatment of N-3 PUFAS on plasma lipoprotein levels and fatty acid composition of total serum and erythrocyte lipids in hypertriglyceridemic patients. *Journal of the Medical Association of Thailand, 88*(2), 181–186.

Spence, L.A., Lipscomb, E.R., Cadogan, J., Martin, B., Wastney, M.E., Peacock, M., et al. (2005). The effect of soy protein and soy isoflavones on calcium metabolism in postmenopausal women: A randomized crossover study. *American Journal of Clinical Nutrition, 81*(4), 916–922.

von Muhlen, D.G., Kritz-Silverstein, D., & Barrett-Connor, E. (1995). A community-based study of menopause symptoms and estrogen replacement in older women. *Maturitas, 22*(2), 71–78.

Chapter 4

American College of Obstetricians and Gynecologists. (2002). ACOG committee opinion. Number 267: Exercise during pregnancy and the postpartum period. *Obstetrics and Gynecology, 99*(1), 171–173.

American College of Sports Medicine (2006). *ACSM's resource manual for guidelines for exercise testing and prescription*. Philadelphia: Lippincott Williams & Wilkins.

Araujo, D. (1997). Expecting questions about exercise and pregnancy? *The Physician and Sportsmedicine, 25*(4), online edition. Retrieved November 7, 2005 from www.physsportsmed.com/issues/1997/4apr/arovjo.htm.

BabyCenter.com (2002, July 20). *Fitness during pregnancy: Pregnancy exercise guide*. Retrieved July 19, 2005 from www.BabyCenter.com.

Ciliberto, C.F., & Marx, G.F. (1998). Physiological changes associated with pregnancy. *Physiology* (9), 1–3.

Kramer, M., & McDonald, S. (2006). Aerobic exercise for women during pregnancy. *Cochrane Database of Systematic Reviews* (3), CD000180.

Mahan, L.K., & Escott-Stump, S. (2004). *Krause's food, nutrition, & diet therapy*. Philadelphia: Saunders (Elsevier).

Mihailov, L. (2002, February 21). I've never exercised before, should I start now? Parenthood.com., online. Retrieved September 16, 2005 from www.pregnancy.parenthood.com.

Orr, T. (1999, July). One size rarely fits all! (Nutrition and metabolism during pregnancy). *Better Nutrition*, online.

Palkhivala, A. (2001, January 18). *Exercise during pregnancy can stimulate baby's growth*. Retrieved October 22, 2006, from www.webmd.com/content/article/18/1676_52365.htm.

Paradise Valley Community College. (2002). *Contraindications to exercise during pregnancy*. Retrieved October 22, 2006, from www.pvc.maricopa.edu/fitness/preg/contraindications.html.

ParentsPlace.com. (2000, November). Another reason to exercise during pregnancy. *Running and Fitness*, Retrieved September 3, 2005 from http://parenting.ivillage.com/pregnancy/pfitness10,,43j2,00.html.

ParentsPlace.com. (2002, July 20). Exercise during pregnancy: Creating a safe and effective workout. *The Women's Network*, online. Retrieved September 8, 2005 from http://parenting.ivillage.com/pregnancy/pfitness10,,43j2,00.html.

Pivarnik, J. (1994). Maternal exercise during pregnancy. *Sports Medicine, 18*(4), 215–217.

Wang, T.W., & Apgar, B.S. (1998). Exercise during pregnancy. *American Family Physician, 57*(8), 1846–1852, 1857.

Chapter 5

Alewaeters, K., Clarys, P., Hebbelinck, M., Deriemaeker, P., & Clarys, J.P. (2005). Cross-sectional analysis of BMI and some lifestyle variables in Flemish vegetarians compared with non-vegetarians. *Ergonomics, 48*(11–14), 1433–1444.

American Dietetic Association and Dietitians of Canada. (2003). Position of the American Dietetic Association and Dietitians of Canada: Vegetarian diets. *Canadian Journal of Dietetic Practice and Research, 64*(2), 62–81.

American Dietetic Association and Dietitians of Canada. (2003). Position of the American Dietetic Association and Dietitians of Canada: Vegetarian diets. *Journal of the American Dietetic Association, 103*(6), 748–765.

Barr, S.I., & Rideout, C.A. (2004). Nutritional considerations for vegetarian athletes. *Nutrition, 20*(7–8), 696–703.

Block, G., Patterson, B., & Subar, A. (1992). Fruit, vegetables, and cancer prevention: A review of the epidemiologic evidence. *Nutrition and Cancer—An International Journal, 18*(1), 1–29.

Dresbach, S., & Rossi, A. (n.d.). *Ohio State University Extension fact sheet*. Retrieved August 1, 2006 from http://ohioline.osu.edu/hyg-fact/5000/5050.html.

Hasler, C.M., Bloch, A.S., Thomson, C.A., Enrione, E., & Manning, C. (2004). Position of the American Dietetic Association: Functional foods. *Journal of the American Dietetic Association, 104*(5), 814–826.

Health Link, Medical College of Wisconsin. (2001, February 13). *Vitamin D*. Retrieved October 25, 2006 from http://healthlink.mcw.edu/article/982088787.html.

Leitzmann, C. (2005). Vegetarian diets: What are the advantages? *Forum Nutrition, 57*, 147–156.

Mangels, R. (2006). *Protein in the vegan diet*. Retrieved October 25, 2006 from Vegetarian Resource Group Web site: www.vrg.org/nutrition/protein.htm.

New Fitness. (n.d.). *Protein—defined, requirements, food source*. Retrieved October 25, 2005 from www.new-fitness.com/nutrition/protein.html.

Polk, M. (1996). Feast on phytochemicals. *American Institute of Cancer Research Newsletter,* issue 51.

Sabate, J. (2003). The contribution of vegetarian diets to human health. *Forum Nutrition, 56*, 218–220.

Thompson, H.J., Heimendinger, J., Diker, A., O'Neill, C., Haegele, A., Meinecke, B., et al. (2006). Dietary botanical diversity affects the reduction of oxidative biomarkers in women due to high vegetable and fruit intake. *Journal of Nutrition, 136*(8), 2207–2212.

U.S. Department of Agriculture, Agricultural Research Service. (1998). *USDA nutrient database for standard reference, release 12.* Retrieved October 25, 2006 from Nutrient Data Laboratory Home Page, www.nal.usda.gov/fnic/foodcomp/Data/SR12/sr12.html.

Veggie Sports Association. (n.d.). *Vegetarian and vegan famous athletes.* Retrieved October 25, 2006 from www.veggie.org/veggie/famous.veg.athletes.shtml.

Vegetarian Society. (n.d.). *Vegetarian information sheet—zinc.* Retrieved October 25, 2006 from http://www.vegsoc.org/info/zinc.html.

Chapter 6

Acheson, K.J., Gremaud, G., Meirim, I., Montigon, F., Krebs, Y., Fay, L.B., et al. (2004). Metabolic effects of caffeine in humans: Lipid oxidation or futile cycling? *American Journal of Clinical Nutrition, 79*(1), 40–46.

Acheson, K.J., Zahorska-Markiewicz, B., Pittet, P., Anantharaman, K., & Jequier, E. (1980). Caffeine and coffee: Their influence on metabolic rate and substrate utilization in normal weight and obese individuals. *American Journal of Clinical Nutrition, 33*(5), 989–997.

Al-Kandari, Y. (2006) Data are for those age 20 and older. www.ncbi.nlm.nih.gov/entrez/query.fcgi?cmd=Retrieve&db=PubMed&dopt=Citation&list_uids=16629871.

Arciero, P.J., Gardner, A.W., Calles-Escandon, J., Benowitz, N.L., & Poehlman, E.T. (1995). Effects of caffeine ingestion on NE kinetics, fat oxidation, and energy expenditure in younger and older men. *American Journal of Physiology, 268*(6 Pt. 1), E1192–1198.

Astrup, A., Toubro, S., Christensen, N.J., & Quaade, F. (1992). Pharmacology of thermogenic drugs. *American Journal of Clinical Nutrition, 55*(1 Suppl.), 246S–248S.

Baumann, G., Felix, S., Sattelberger, U., & Klein, G. (1990). Cardiovascular effects of forskolin (HL 362) in patients with idiopathic congestive cardiomyopathy—a comparative study with dobutamine and sodium nitroprusside. *Journal of Cardiovascular Pharmacology, 16*(1), 93–100.

Bellet, S., Roman, L., DeCastro, O., Kim, K.E., & Kershbaum, A. (1969). Effect of coffee ingestion on catecholamine release. *Metabolism, 18*(4), 288–291.

Bent, S., Padula, A., & Neuhaus, J. (2004). Safety and efficacy of citrus aurantium for weight loss. *American Journal of Cardiology, 94*(10), 1359–1361.

Blair, S.N., Kohl, H.W., 3rd, Paffenbarger, R.S., Jr., Clark, D.G., Cooper, K.H., & Gibbons, L.W. (1989). Physical fitness and all-cause mortality. A prospective study of healthy men and women. *Journal of the American Medical Association, 262*(17), 2395–2401.

Booth, S.L., Madabushi, H.T., Davidson, K.W., & Sadowski, J.A. (1995). Tea and coffee brews are not dietary sources of vitamin K-1 (phylloquinone). *Journal of the American Dietetic Association, 95*(1), 82–83.

Boutelle, K.N., & Kirschenbaum, D.S. (1998). Further support for consistent self-monitoring as a vital component of successful weight control. *Obesity Research, 6*(3), 219–224.

Bracco, D., Ferrarra, J.M., Arnaud, M.J., Jequier, E., & Schutz, Y. (1995). Effects of caffeine on energy metabolism, heart rate, and methylxanthine metabolism in lean and obese women. *American Journal of Physiology, 269*(4 Pt. 1), E671–678.

Bryner, R.W., Ullrich, I.H., Sauers, J., Donley, D., Hornsby, G., Kolar, M., et al. (1999). Effects of resistance vs. aerobic training combined with an 800 calorie liquid diet on lean body mass and resting metabolic rate. *Journal of the American College of Nutrition, 18*(2), 115–121.

Butcher, R.W., Baird, C.E., & Sutherland, E.W. (1968). Effects of lipolytic and antilipolytic substances on adenosine 3',5'-monophosphate levels in isolated fat cells. *Journal of Biological Chemistry, 243*(8), 1705–1712.

Chantre, P., & Lairon, D. (2002). Recent findings of green tea extract AR25 (Exolise) and its activity for the treatment of obesity. *Phytomedicine, 9*(1), 3–8.

Daly, J.M., Heymsfield, S.B., Head, C.A., Harvey, L.P., Nixon, D.W., Katzeff, H., et al. (1985). Human energy requirements: Overestimation by widely used prediction equation. *American Journal of Clinical Nutrition, 42*(6), 1170–1174.

Danforth, E., Jr. (1985). Diet and obesity. *American Journal of Clinical Nutrition, 41*(5 Suppl.), 1132–1145.

Davi, G., Guagnano, M.T., Ciabattoni, G., Basili, S., Falco, A., Marinopiccoli, M., et al. (2002). Platelet activation in obese women: Role of inflammation and oxidant stress. *Journal of the American Medical Association, 288*(16), 2008–2014.

Debrah, K., Haigh, R., Sherwin, R., Murphy, J., & Kerr, D. (1995). Effect of acute and chronic caffeine use on the cerebrovascular, cardiovascular and hormonal responses to orthostasis in healthy volunteers. *Clinical Science (London), 89*(5), 475–480.

Diepvens, K., Kovacs, E.M., Nijs, I.M., Vogels, N., & Westerterp-Plantenga, M.S. (2005). Effect of green tea on resting energy expenditure and substrate oxidation during weight loss in overweight females. *British Journal of Nutrition, 94*(6), 1026–1034.

Donnelly, J.E., Sharp, T., Houmard, J., Carlson, M.G., Hill, J.O., Whatley, J.E., et al. (1993). Muscle hypertrophy with large-scale weight loss and resistance training. *American Journal of Clinical Nutrition, 58*(4), 561–565.

Dulloo, A.G., Duret, C., Rohrer, D., Girardier, L., Mensi, N., Fathi, M., et al. (1999). Efficacy of a green tea extract rich in catechin polyphenols and caffeine in increasing 24-h energy expenditure and fat oxidation in humans. *American Journal of Clinical Nutrition, 70*(6), 1040–1045.

Dyck, D.J. (2000). Dietary fat intake, supplements, and weight loss. *Canadian Journal of Applied Physiology, 25*(6), 495–523.

Federal Trade Commission. (2002). *Weight-loss advertising: An analysis of current trends.*

Filozof, C., Gonzalez, C., Sereday, M., Mazza, C., & Braguinsky, J. (2001). Obesity prevalence and trends in Latin-American countries. *Obesity Reviews, 2*(2), 99–106.

Food and Nutrition Board of the Institute of Medicine. Panel on Macronutrients, Standing Committee on the Scientific Evaluation of Dietary Reference Intakes. (2005). *Dietary reference intakes for energy, carbohydrate, fiber, fat, fatty acids, cholesterol, protein, and amino acids.* Washington, DC: National Academy Press.

Food and Nutrition Board of the Institute of Medicine. Standing Committee on the Scientific Evaluation of Dietary Reference Intakes. (1997). *Dietary reference intakes for calcium, phosphorus, magnesium, vitamin D, and fluoride.* Washington, DC: National Academy Press.

Food and Nutrition Board of the Institute of Medicine. Standing Committee on the Scientific Evaluation of Dietary Reference Intakes. Panel on Folate, Other B Vitamins, and Choline. Subcommittee on Upper Reference Levels of Nutrients. (1998). *Dietary reference intakes for thiamin, riboflavin, niacin, vitamin B_6, folate, vitamin B_{12}, pantothenic acid, biotin, and choline.* Washington, DC: National Academy Press.

Frankenfield, D., Roth-Yousey, L., & Compher, C. (2005). Comparison of predictive equations for resting metabolic rate in healthy nonobese and obese adults: A systematic review. *Journal of the American Dietetic Association, 105*(5), 775–789.

Gades, M.D., & Stern, J.S. (2005). Chitosan supplementation and fat absorption in men and women. *Journal of the American Dietetic Association, 105*(1), 72–77.

Geliebter, A., Maher, M.M., Gerace, L., Gutin, B., Heymsfield, S.B., & Hashim, S.A. (1997). Effects of strength or aerobic training on body composition, resting metabolic rate, and peak oxygen consumption in obese dieting subjects. *American Journal of Clinical Nutrition, 66*(3), 557–563.

Godard, M.P., Johnson, B.A., & Richmond, S.R. (August 2005). Body composition and hormonal adaptations associated with forskolin consumption in overweight and obese men. *Obes. Res. 13*(8): 1335-1343.

Guerciolini, R., Radu-Radulescu, L., Boldrin, M., Dallas, J., & Moore, R. (2001). Comparative evaluation of fecal fat excretion induced by orlistat and chitosan. *Obesity Research, 9*(6), 364–367.

Haaz, S., Fontaine, K.R., Cutter, G., Limdi, N., Perumean-Chaney, S., & Allison, D.B. (2006). Citrus aurantium and synephrine alkaloids in the treatment of overweight and obesity: An update. *Obesity Reviews, 7*(1), 79–88.

Han, L.K., Morimoto, C., Yu, R.H., & Okuda, H. (2005). Effects of Coleus forskohlii on fat storage in ovariectomized rats. *Yakugaku Zasshi, 125*(5), 449–453.

Harris, J.A., & Benedict, F.G. (1919). *A biometric study of basal metabolism in man.* Washington, DC: Carnegie Institution of Washington.

Hedley, A.A., Ogden, C.L., Johnson, C.L., Carroll, M.D., Curtin, L.R., & Flegal, K.M. (2004). Prevalence of overweight and obesity among US children, adolescents, and adults, 1999-2002. *Journal of the American Medical Association, 291*(23), 2847-2850.

Hellerstein, M.K. (1998). Is chromium supplementation effective in managing type II diabetes? *Nutrition Reviews, 56*(10), 302-306.

Heymsfield, S.B., Darby, P.C., Muhlheim, L.S., Gallagher, D., Wolper, C., & Allison, D.B. (1995). The calorie: Myth, measurement, and reality. *American Journal of Clinical Nutrition, 62*(5 Suppl.), 1034S-1041S.

Horton, E.S. (1983). Introduction: An overview of the assessment and regulation of energy balance in humans. *American Journal of Clinical Nutrition, 38*(6), 972-977.

Jakicic, J.M. (2003a). Exercise in the treatment of obesity. *Endocrinology and Metabolism Clinics of North America, 32*(4), 967-980.

Jakicic, J.M. (2003b). Exercise strategies for the obese patient. *Primary Care, 30*(2), 393-403.

Jakicic, J.M., Clark, K., Coleman, E., Donnelly, J.E., Foreyt, J., Melanson, E., et al. (2001). American College of Sports Medicine position stand. Appropriate intervention strategies for weight loss and prevention of weight regain for adults. *Medicine and Science in Sports and Exercise, 33*(12), 2145-2156.

Jakicic, J.M., Wing, R.R., Butler, B.A., & Robertson, R.J. (1995). Prescribing exercise in multiple short bouts versus one continuous bout: Effects on adherence, cardiorespiratory fitness, and weight loss in overweight women. *International Journal of Obesity and Related Metabolic Disorders, 19*(12), 893-901.

Kreider, R., S. Henderson, B. Maghu, C. Rasmussen, S. Lancaster, C. Kerksick, P. Smith, C. Melton, P. Cowan, M. Greenwood, C. Earnest, A. Almada, & P. Milnor. (2002). Effects of coleus forskohlii supplementation on body composition and markers of health in sedentary overweight females. FASEB Journal, 16, LB59.

King, A.C., Haskell, W.L., Taylor, C.B., Kraemer, H.C., & DeBusk, R.F. (1991). Group- vs home-based exercise training in healthy older men and women. A community-based clinical trial. *Journal of the American Medical Association, 266*(11), 1535-1542.

Kopelman, P.G. (2000). Obesity as a medical problem. *Nature, 404*(6778), 635-643.

Kotz, C.M., & Levine, J.A. (2005). Role of non-exercise activity thermogenesis (NEAT) in obesity. *Minnesota Medicine, 88*(9), 54-57.

Ledikwe, J.H., Ello-Martin, J.A., & Rolls, B.J. (2005). Portion sizes and the obesity epidemic. *Journal of Nutrition, 135*(4), 905-909.

Levine, J.A., Lanningham-Foster, L.M., McCrady, S.K., Krizan, A.C., Olson, L.R., Kane, P.H., et al. (2005). Interindividual variation in posture allocation: Possible role in human obesity. *Science, 307*(5709), 584-586.

Malpuech-Brugere, C., Verboeket-van de Venne, W.P., Mensink, R.P., Arnal, M.A., Morio, B., Brandolini, M., et al. (2004). Effects of two conjugated linoleic acid isomers on body fat mass in overweight humans. *Obesity Research, 12*(4), 591-598.

Mattes, R.D., & Bormann, L. (2000). Effects of (-)-hydroxycitric acid on appetitive variables. *Physiology and Behavior, 71*(1-2), 87-94.

Mhurchu, C.N., Dunshea-Mooij, C.A., Bennett, D., & Rodgers, A. (2005a). Effect of chitosan on weight loss in overweight and obese individuals: A systematic review of randomized controlled trials. *Obesity Reviews, 6*(1), 35-42.

Mhurchu, C.N., Dunshea-Mooij, C.A., Bennett, D., & Rodgers, A. (2005b). Chitosan for overweight or obesity. *Cochrane Database of Systematic Reviews* (3), CD003892.

Mhurchu, C.N., Poppitt, S.D., McGill, A.T., Leahy, F.E., Bennett, D.A., Lin, R.B., et al. (2004). The effect of the dietary supplement, chitosan, on body weight: A randomised controlled trial in 250 overweight and obese adults. *International Journal of Obesity and Related Metabolic Disorders, 28*(9), 1149-1156.

Mifflin, M.D., St. Jeor, S.T., Hill, L.A., Scott, B.J., Daugherty, S.A., & Koh, Y.O. (1990). A new predictive equation for resting energy expenditure in healthy individuals. *American Journal of Clinical Nutrition, 51*(2), 241-247.

Mokhtar, N., Elati, J., Chabir, R., Bour, A., Elkari, K., Schlossman, N.P., Caballero, B., and Aguenaou, H. Diet culture and obesity in northern Africa. J Nutrition 2001. 131:887S-892S. www.ncbi.nlm.nih.gov/entrez/query.fcgi?cmd=Retrieve&db=PubMed&dopt=Citation&list_uids=11238780.

Mutlu, G.M., Koch, W.J., & Factor, P. (2004). Alveolar epithelial β_2-adrenergic receptors: Their role in regulation of alveolar active sodium transport. *American Journal of Respiratory and Critical Care Medicine, 170,* 1270–1275.

National Heart, Lung, and Blood Institute (NHLBI), a division of the National Institutes of Health. www.nhlbi.nih.gov

Novak, C.M., Zhang, M., & Levine, J.A. (2006). Neuromedin u in the paraventricular and arcuate hypothalamic nuclei increases non-exercise activity thermogenesis. *Journal of Neuroendocrinology, 18*(8), 594–601.

Ogden, C.L., Carroll, M.D., Curtin L.R., McDowell, M.A., Tabak, C.J., & Flegal, K.M. (2006). Prevalence of overweight and obesity in the United States, 1999–2004. *Journal of the American Medical Association, 295*(13), 1549–1555.

Pariza, M.W., & Ha, Y.L. (1990). Conjugated dienoic derivatives of linoleic acid: A new class of anticarcinogens. *Medical Oncology and Tumor Pharmacotherapy, 7*(2–3), 169–171.

Pereira, M.A., Parker, E.D., & Folsom, A.R. (2006). Coffee consumption and risk of type 2 diabetes mellitus: An 11-year prospective study of 28,812 postmenopausal women. *Archives of Internal Medicine, 166*(12), 1311–1316.

Perri, M.G. (1998). The maintenance of treatment effects in the long-term management of obesity. *Clinical Psychology: Science and Practice, 5,* 526–543.

Perri, M.G., Martin, A.D., Leermakers, E.A., Sears, S.F., & Notelovitz, M. (1997). Effects of group- versus home-based exercise in the treatment of obesity. *Journal of Consulting and Clinical Psychology, 65*(2), 278–285.

Pittler, M.H., & Ernst, E. (2004). Dietary supplements for body-weight reduction: A systematic review. *American Journal of Clinical Nutrition, 79*(4), 529–536.

Ravussin, E., & Bogardus, C. (1992). A brief overview of human energy metabolism and its relationship to essential obesity. *American Journal of Clinical Nutrition, 55*(1 Suppl.), 242S–245S.

Riserus, U., Smedman, A., Basu, S., & Vessby, B. (2003). CLA and body weight regulation in humans. *Lipids, 38*(2), 133–137.

Riserus, U., Vessby, B., Arnlov, J., & Basu, S. (2004). Effects of cis-9,trans-11 conjugated linoleic acid supplementation on insulin sensitivity, lipid peroxidation, and proinflammatory markers in obese men.

American Journal of Clinical Nutrition, 80(2), 279–283.

Ritzenthaler, K.L., McGuire, M.K., Falen, R., Shultz, T.D., Dasgupta, N., & McGuire, M.A. (2001). Estimation of conjugated linoleic acid intake by written dietary assessment methodologies underestimates actual intake evaluated by food duplicate methodology. *Journal of Nutrition, 131*(5), 1548–1554.

Son, D.J., Cho, M.R., Jin, Y.R., Kim, S.Y., Park, Y.H., Lee, S.H., et al. (2004). Antiplatelet effect of green tea catechins: A possible mechanism through arachidonic acid pathway. *Prostaglandins, Leukotrienes and Essential Fatty Acids, 71*(1), 25–31.

Taylor, J.R., & Wilt, V.M. (1999). Probable antagonism of warfarin by green tea. *Annals of Pharmacotherapy, 33*(4), 426–428.

Terpstra, A.H. (2004). Effect of conjugated linoleic acid on body composition and plasma lipids in humans: An overview of the literature. *American Journal of Clinical Nutrition, 79*(3), 352–361.

U.S. Department of Agriculture and U.S. Department of Health and Human Services. (2005). *Dietary Guidelines for Americans 2005* (6th ed.). Washington, DC.

van Loon, L.J., van Rooijen, J.J., Niesen, B., Verhagen, H., Saris, W.H., & Wagenmakers, A.J. (2000). Effects of acute (-)-hydroxycitrate supplementation on substrate metabolism at rest and during exercise in humans. *American Journal of Clinical Nutrition, 72*(6), 1445–1450.

Villani, R.G., Gannon, J., Self, M., & Rich, P.A. (2000). L-Carnitine supplementation combined with aerobic training does not promote weight loss in moderately obese women. *International Journal of Sport Nutrition and Exercise Metabolism, 10*(2), 199–207.

Volpe, S.L., Huang, H.W., Larpadisorn, K., & Lesser, I.I. (2001). Effect of chromium supplementation and exercise on body composition, resting metabolic rate and selected biochemical parameters in moderately obese women following an exercise program. *Journal of the American College of Nutrition, 20*(4), 293–306.

Wadden, T.A., Vogt, R.A., Andersen, R.E., Bartlett, S.J., Foster, G.D., Kuehnel, R.H., et al. (1997). Exercise in the treatment of obesity: Effects of four interventions on body composition, resting energy expenditure, appetite, and mood. *Journal of Consulting and Clinical Psychology, 65*(2), 269–277.

World Health Organization (1997). *Obesity: Preventing and Managing the Global Epidemic—Report of a WHO Consultation on Obesity.* Geneva, June 3–5

Wu, C.H., Lu, F.H., Chang, C.S., Chang, T.C., Wang, R.H., & Chang, C.J. (2003). Relationship among habitual tea consumption, percent body fat, and body fat distribution. *Obesity Research, 11*(9), 1088–1095.

Chapter 7

Alberti, K.G., & Zimmet, P.Z. (1998). Definition, diagnosis and classification of diabetes mellitus and its complications. Part 1: Diagnosis and classification of diabetes mellitus. Provisional report of a WHO consultation. *Diabetic Medicine, 15*(7), 539–553.

American Diabetes Association. (2003). Report of the Expert Committee on the Diagnosis and Classification of Diabetes Mellitus. *Diabetes Care, 26*, S5–S20.

American Diabetes Association. (2004). Physical activity/exercise and diabetes. *Diabetes Care, 27*, S58–S62.

Boule, N.G., Haddard, E., Kenny, G.P., Wells, G.A., & Sigal R.J. (2001). Effects of exercise on glycemic control and body mass in type 2 diabetes mellitus: A meta-analysis of controlled clinical trials. *Journal of the American Medical Association, 286*(10), 1218–1227.

Colberg, S. (2001). *The diabetic athlete: Prescriptions for exercise and sport.* Champaign, IL: Human Kinetics.

Expert Panel on Detection, Evaluation, and Treatment of High Blood Cholesterol in Adults. (2001). Executive Summary of the Third Report of the National Cholesterol Education Program (NCEP). *Journal of the American Medical Association, 285*, 2486–2497.

Foster, G.D., Wyatt, H.R., Hill, J.O., McGuckin, B.G., Brill, C., Mohammed, B.S., et al. (2003). A randomized trial of a low-carbohydrate diet for obesity. *New England Journal of Medicine, 348*(21), 2082–2090.

Goss, J.A., Schock, A.P., Brunicardi, F.C., Goodpastor, S.E., Garber, A.J., Soltes, G., et al. (2002). Achievement of insulin independence in three consecutive type-1 diabetic patients via pancreatic islet transplantation using islets isolated at a remote islet isolation center. *Transplantation, 74*(12), 1761–1766.

Gupta, A., Gupta, R., Sarna, M., Rastogi, S., Gupta, V.P., & Kothari, K. (2003). Prevalence of diabetes, impaired fasting glucose and insulin resistance syndrome in an urban Indian population. *Diabetes Research in Clinical Practice, 61*(1), 69–76.

Horton, E. (1998). Role and management of exercise in diabetes mellitus. *Diabetes Care,* 11(2), 201–211.

Hu, F.B., Sigal, R.J., Rich-Edwards, J.W., Colditz, G.A., Solomon, C.G., Willett, W.C., et al. (1991). Walking compared with vigorous physical activity and risk of type 2 diabetes in women: A prospective study. *Journal of the American Medical Association, 282*(15), 1433–1439.

Jakicic, J.M., Winters, C., Lang, W., & Wing, R. (1999). Effects of intermittent exercise and use of home-exercise equipment on adherence, weight loss, and fitness in overweight women. A randomized trial. *Journal of the American Medical Association, 282*, 1554–1560.

Laaksonen, D.E., Lakka, H.M., Niskanen, L.K., Kaplan, G.A., Salonen, J.T., & Lakka, T.A. (2002). Metabolic syndrome and development of diabetes mellitus: Application and validation of recently suggested definitions of the metabolic syndrome in a prospective cohort study. *American Journal of Epidemiology, 156*(11), 1070–1077.

Lee, W.Y., Park, J.S., Noh, S.Y., Rhee, E.J., Kim, S.W., & Zimmet, P.Z. (2004). Prevalence of the metabolic syndrome among 40,698 Korean metropolitan subjects. *Diabetes Research in Clinical Practice, 65*(2),143–149.

Pettitt, D. (1998). Gestational diabetes mellitus: Who to test. How to test. *Diabetes Care,* 21(11), 1789.

Rennie, K.L., McCarthy, N., Yazdgerdi, S., Marmot, M., & Brunner, E. (2003). Association of the metabolic syndrome with both vigorous and moderate physical activity. *International Journal of Epidemiology,* 32(4), 600–606.

Rybka, J. (1987). Diabetes mellitus and exercise. *Acta Universitatis Carolinae Medica Monographs, 118*, 1–133.

Sargrad, K.R., Homko, C., Mozzoli, M., & Boden, G. (2005). Effect of high protein vs high carbohydrate intake on insulin sensitivity, body weight, hemoglobin A1c, and blood pressure in patients with type 2 diabetes mellitus. *Journal of the American Dietetic Association, 105*(4), 573–580.

Sattar, N., Gaw, A., Scherbakova, O., Ford, I., O'Reilly, D.S., Haffner, S.M., et al. (2003). Metabolic syndrome with and without C-reactive protein as a predictor of coronary heart disease and diabetes in the West of Scotland Coronary Prevention Study. *Circulation, 108*(4), 414–419.

Schneider, S.H., Khachadurian, A.K., Amorosa, L.F., Clemow, L., & Ruderman, N.B. (1992). Ten-year experience with an exercise-based outpatient life-style modification program in the treatment of diabetes mellitus. *Diabetes Care, 14*(11), 1800–1810.

Trucco, M. (2006). Is facilitating pancreatic beta cell regeneration a valid option for clinical therapy? *Cell Transplantation, 15*(Suppl. 1), S75–S84.

Villegas, R., Perry, I.J., Creagh, D., Hinchion, R., & O'Halloran, D. (2003). Prevalence of the metabolic syndrome in middle-aged men and women. *Diabetes Care, 26*(11), 3198–3199.

Walsh, J., & Roberts, R. (1994). *Pumping insulin: Everything in a book for successful use of an insulin pump* (2nd ed.). San Diego: Torrey Pines Press.

World Health Organization. (2000). Retrieved August 8, 2006 from www.who.int/diabetes/facts/world_figures/en/index.html.

Chapter 8

American Psychiatric Association. (2000). Practice guideline for the treatment of patients with eating disorders (revision). *American Journal of Psychiatry, 157*(1 Suppl.), 1–39.

Andersen, A. (1992). Eating disorders in male athletes: A special case? In K.D. Brownell, J. Rodin, & J.H. Wilmore (Eds.), *Eating, body weight and performance in athletes: Disorders of modern society* (pp. 172–188). Philadelphia: Lea and Febiger.

Andersen, A. (1995). Eating disorders in males. In C. Fairburn & K.D. Brownell (Eds.), *Eating disorders and obesity: A comprehensive handbook* (pp. 177–187). New York: Guilford Press.

Beals, K.A. (2004). *Disordered eating among athletes: A comprehensive guide for health professionals.* Champaign, IL: Human Kinetics.

Bruce, B., & Agras, W.S. (1992). Binge eating in females: A population-based investigation. *International Journal of Eating Disorders, 12,* 365–373.

Byrne, S., & McLean, N. (2001). Eating disorders in athletes: A review of the literature. *Journal of Science and Medicine in Sport,* 2001(4): 145-159.

Hobart, J.A., & Smucker, D. (2000). The female athlete triad. *American Family Physician, 61*(11). Retrieved November 5, 2006 from www.aafp.org/afp/20000601/3357.html.

Horton, E. (1988). Role and management of exercise in diabetes mellitus. *Diabetes Care, 11*(2), 201–211.

Kreipe, R.E., & Bindorf, S.A. (2000). Eating disorders in adolescents and young adults. *Medical Clinics of North America, 84,* 1027–1049.

National Institute of Mental Health. (2001). *Eating disorders: Facts about eating disorders and the search for solutions.* Retrieved November 3, 2006 from www.nimh.nih.gov/publicat/eatingdisorders.cfm#intro.

Office on Women's Health, U.S. Department of Health and Human Services. (2000). *Eating disorders.* Retrieved November 29, 2005 from www.4woman.gov/owh/pub/factsheets/eatingdis.htm.

Otis C.L., Drinkwater, B., Johnson, M., Loucks, A., & Wilmore, J. (1997). American College of Sports Medicine position stand: The female athlete triad. *Medicine and Science in Sports and Exercise, 29*(5), i–ix.

Pritts, S.D., & Sussman, J. (2003). Diagnosis of eating disorders in primary care. *American Family Physician, 67*(2), 297–304, 311–312.

Spitzer, R.L., Yanovski, S., Wadden, T., Wing, R., Marcus, M.D., Stunkard, A., et al. (1993). Binge eating disorder: Its further validation in a multisite study. *International Journal of Eating Disorders, 13*(2), 137–153.

Woolsey, M.M. (2002). *Eating disorders: A clinical guide to counseling and treatment.* Chicago: American Dietetic Association.

Yeager, K.K, Agostini, R., Nattiv, A., & Drinkwater, B. (1993). The female athlete triad. *Medicine and Science in Sports and Exercise, 25*, 775–777.

Chapter 9

American College of Sports Medicine (ACSM). (2005, July 26). Guidance to athletes on preventing hyponatremia and dehydration during upcoming races. Newly published roundtable statement on hydration and physical activity reinforces importance of managing both conditions. [News release].

American College of Sports Medicine. Position Stand: Prevention of cold injuries during exercise. (2006). Medicine and Science in Sports and Exercise, 38(11): 2012-2029.

Binkley, H.M., Beckett, J., Casa, D.J., Kleiner, D.M., & Plummer, P.E. (2002). National Athletic Trainers' Association position statement: Exertional heat illnesses. *Journal of Athletic Training, 37*, 329–343.

Burruss, P., Castellani, J., Rundell, K., & Snyder, A. (1998). Roundtable: Winter sports. Gatorade Sports Science Institute.

Butterfield, G., Gates, J., Fleming, S., Brooks, G.A., Sutton, J.R., & Reeves, J.T. (1992). Increased energy intake minimizes weight loss in men at high altitude. *Journal of Applied Physiology, 72*, 1741–1768.

Casa, D. (2002). Preventing exertional heat illness: A consensus statement. *GSSI Sports Science News.* Gatorade Sports Science Institute.

Fein, L.W., Haymes, E.M., & Buskirk, E.R. (1975). Effects of daily and intermittent exposure on heat acclimation of women. *International Journal of Biometeorology, 19*, 41–52.

Gore Trail Condominiums (2002). *High altitude information.* Retrieved November 10, 2005, from www.goretrail.com/altitude.html

Green, H.J., Sutton, J.R., Young, P.M., Cymerman, A., & Houston, C.S. (1989). Operation Everest II: Muscle energetics during maximal exhaustive exercise. *Journal of Applied Physiology, 66*, 142–150.

Hargreaves, M. (1996). Exercise performance in the heat. *Gatorade Sports Science Exchange, 2*(1).

Houmard, J.A., Costill, D.L., Davis, J.A., Mitchell, J.B., Pascoe, D.D., & Robergs, R.A. (1990). The influence of exercise intensity on heat acclimation in trained subjects. *Medicine and Science in Sports and Exercise, 22*, 615–620.

Kreider, R., Greenwood, M., Greenwood, L., & Leutholtz, B. (2003, May). Ephedra update: Ephedra blamed for contributing to death of a major league baseball player. *Muscular Development*, 150–153.

Lind, A.R., & Bass, D.E. (1963). Optimal exposure time for development of heat acclimation. *Federation Proceedings, 22*, 704–708.

MacDougall, J.D., Green, H.J., Sutton, J.R., Coates, G., Cymerman, A., Young, P., et al. (1991). Operation Everest II: Structural adaptations in skeletal muscle in response to extreme simulated altitude. *Acta Physiologica Scandinavia, 142*, 421–427.

Maughan, R.J., & Shirreffs, S. (1997). Preparing athletes for competition in the heat: Developing an effective acclimization strategy. *Gatorade Sports Science Exchange, 10*(2).

Murray, R. (1996). Preventing dehydration and hyperthermia. *Gatorade Sports Science Exchange, 2*(1).

Murray, R. (2002). How often should you drink fluids? *Gatorade Sports Science Exchange.* Retrieved from www.gssiweb.org.

Murray, R. (2005). Preventing dehydration: Sports drinks or water. *Gatorade Sports Science Exchange.* Retrieved from www.gssiweb.org.

Pichan, G., Sridharan, K., Swamy, Y.V., Joseph, S., & Gautam, R.K. (1985). Physiological acclimatization to heat after a spell of cold conditioning in tropical subjects. *Aviation, Space and Environmental Medicine, 56*, 436–440.

Sawka, M.N., & Pandolf, K. (1990). Effects of body water loss on physiological function and exercise performance. In C.V. Gisolfi & D.R. Lamb (Eds.), *Perspectives in exercise science and sports medicine. Vol. 3. Fluid homeostasis during exercise* (pp. 1–38). Indianapolis: Benchmark Press.

SurvivalIQ. (2003). Retrieved November 10, 2006, from www.survivaliq.com/index.htm

Sutton, J. (1993). Exercise training at high altitude: Does it improve endurance performance at sea level? *Gatorade Sports Science Exchange, 6*(4).

Sutton, J. (1996). Heat acclimatisation. *Gatorade Sports Science Exchange, 2*(1).

Index

Note: The italicized *f* and *t* following page numbers refer to figures and tables, respectively.

About the Authors

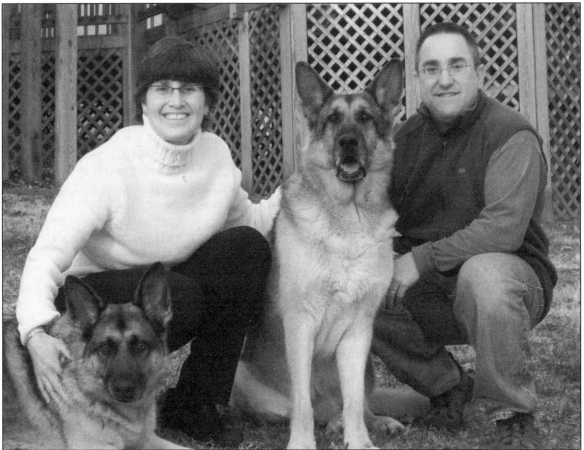

Courtesy of May May Leung

Stella Lucia Volpe, PhD, RD, LDN, FACSM, is associate professor and the Miriam Stirl Term endowed chair of nutrition at the University of Pennsylvania School of Nursing, Division of Biobehavioral and Health Sciences. She is certified by the American College of Sports Medicine as an exercise specialist and is a registered and licensed dietitian. Her research in sport nutrition and obesity prevention spans more than 15 years.

She is a fellow of the American College of Sports Medicine and a member of the American Dietetic Association; its dietetic practice group, SCAN (Sports, Cardiovascular, and Wellness Nutritionists); and the American Society for Nutrition. She

won the University Distinguished Teaching Award at the University of Massachusetts at Amherst. Dr. Volpe holds a bachelor's degree in exercise physiology from the University of Pittsburgh as well as a master's degree in exercise physiology and a doctorate in nutrition, both from Virginia Tech.

Dr. Volpe is an avid exerciser and a life-long athlete. She has completed numerous road races (of varying distances), triathlons, and a marathon. She is a competitive rower and field hockey player; performs Pilates, yoga, and kickboxing; and lifts weights. Dr. Volpe especially enjoys cross-country skiing, snowshoeing, and hiking with her husband and German shepherd dogs.

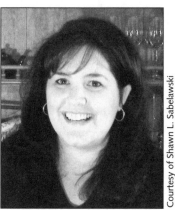

Courtesy of Shawn L. Sabelawski

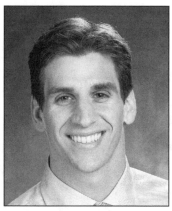

Courtesy of Alliance Photography Group

Sara Bernier Sabelawski, MEd, RD, LDN, is a lecturer, undergraduate program director, and director of the didactic program in dietetics at the University of Massachusetts at Amherst. She is a registered and licensed dietitian and has worked with many populations and various disease states, including pregnant women, people with diabetes, postmenopausal women, and people with eating disorders and weight management issues. She is a member of the American Dietetic Association and the American Society of Parenteral and Enteral Nutrition. She enjoys various kinds of activities such as cardiovascular exercise, weight training, swimming, and yoga. She particularly enjoys outdoor activities like biking, hiking, snowshoeing, and downhill and cross-country skiing.

Christopher R. Mohr, PhD, RD, CSSD, is president of Mohr Results, Inc, a fitness and nutrition consulting company. He has worked with all levels of athletes, from high school to professionals. He was a sport nutritionist at the University of Massachusetts at Amherst and is currently a nutrition consultant to the University of Louisville athletics program. He is a registered dietitian and a board-certified specialist in sport dietetics. Dr. Mohr is a member of the American College of Sports Medicine, American Dietetic Association, and SCAN (Sports, Cardiovascular, and Wellness Nutritionists). He earned a bachelor's degree in nutrition from Pennsylvania State University, a master's degree in nutrition from the University of Massachusetts at Amherst, and a PhD in exercise physiology from the University of Pittsburgh.

Dr. Mohr is an exercise enthusiast. He has been a competitive athlete throughout his life, and currently enjoys weight training, cycling, cross-country skiing, and virtually any other outdoor activity.